The Premier Advance

(MCQ's for Post Graduation Unani Entrance Examination)

By

Dr **Izharul Hasan** MD (Unani)
Dr **Shah Faisal** MD (Unani)
Dr **Danish K Chishti** MD (Unani)

Academic Independent Publishing Platform,
South Carolina, North Charleston, USA

Co-authors and designed by:

Dr. Rehnuma Parveen

B.U.M.S from Ayurvedic & Unani Tibbia College, Karol Bagh, University of Delhi in 2012

M.D (Moalajat) from Jamia Tibbiya Deoband, CCS University of Meerut (Batch 2015-16)

Dr. Junaid Nazir Dandroo MS (Unani)

B.U.M.S from Ayurvedic & Unani Tibbia College, Karol Bagh, University of Delhi in 2014

House surgeon from Ayurvedic & Unani Tibbia College, Karol Bagh, University of Delhi in 2014

M.S (Unani) from National Institute of Unani Medicine, Bangalore (Batch 2015-16)

Book Details

Paperback: 276 pages
Publisher: Academic Independent Publishing Platform; 1st edition (March, 2017), 2nd Ed Nov 2019
ISBN-10: 1545150451
ISBN-13: 978-1545150450
Product Dimensions: 6 x 9 inches

drizharulhasan@2016-17 by publishing platform and author

All rights reserved@Dr Izharul Hasan

No part of this publication may be reproduced or transmitted in any form or by any means, electronic, mechanical, photocopy, recording, translated, or any information storage and retrieval system, without permission in writing from the publishing platform and author.

This book has been published in good faith that the material provided by editor/author(s) contained herein is original, and is intended for educational/personal purposes only. Every effort is made to ensure accuracy of material, but publisher and printing platform will not be held responsible for any inadvertent errors, liability, or loss incurred, directly or indirectly, from the use or application of any of the contents of this work. If not specifically stated, all figures and tables are courtesy of the author.

Corresponding email: drizharnium@gmail.com

Contact: 91-8287833547
The Premier Advance
First Edition: Ed 2017, 2nd Ed 2019
Publisher: Academic Independent Publishing Platform; 2nd edition

PREFACE

We are indeed gratified by the students, teachers and institutions response to our previous books entitled as **"The Prime": Mcqs for Post Graduation Unani Entrance Examination (more than 4000 mcq's with answer key) and "The Premier", Previous Examination Papers of MD Unani Amu Aligarh (2300 mcq's with answer key) by Dr Izharul Hasan and Dr Haqeeq Ahmad.** It is pride and pleasure that we place the new book entitled **"The Premier Advance"**.

The main features of the book are as follows:

- ❖ The book is designed exclusively as per the MCQ pattern of examination prescribed by NIUM and AMU for PG Unani Entrance examination.
- ❖ 1,000 MCQs has been given PG entrance examination as well as test your knowledge with Key answers.
- ❖ Test your knowledge papers are given for the practice of the students so that they can gain confidence for actual exam.
- ❖ Latest exam papers are given along with answers.

We are thankful to our students who gave us encouragement to present this book. We shall be grateful for any of your suggestion to improve the book further. The team of authors would like to receive compliments, comments or criticism from you. We owe a debt of gratitude to all our worthy readers for their overwhelming acceptance and valuable suggestions. Suggestions regarding the subject matter and the pattern shall be welcomed. These may be sent to authors through the publisher or directly by email at drizharnium@gmail.com. We are also thankful to academic publication and their staff for their co-operation in presenting the book to students online all over India.

We thank you, one and all.

ACKNOWLEDGEMENT

First and foremost, I have to thank my parents for their love and support throughout my life. Thank you both for giving me strength to reach the stars and chase my dreams. My brothers, sisters, and other family members deserve my wholehearted thanks as well.

I would like to express my gratitude to the many people who saw me through this book; to all those who provided support, talked things over, read, wrote, offered comments, allowed me to quote their remarks and assisted in the editing, proofreading and design.

I would like to thank my wife for standing beside me throughout my career and writing this book. She has been my inspiration and motivation for continuing to improve my knowledge and move my career forward.

I would like to thanks my all friends for understanding and encouragement in my many, many moments of crisis. Your friendship makes my life a wonderful experience. I cannot list all the names here, but you are always on my mind.

Once again thanks my parents and family members, for sharing my happiness when starting this book and following with encouragement when it seemed too difficult to be completed. I would have probably give up without their support and example on what to do when you really want something.

Thank you, Lord, for always being there for me.

Izharul Hasan

INDEX

SN	Title	Page No.
1	NIUM ENTRANCE EXAMINATION 2014	9-30
2	NIUM ENTRANCE EXAMINATION 2015	31-52
3	NIUM ENTRANCE EXAMINATION 2016	53-74
4	AMU ENTRANCE EXAMINATION FOR PG UNANI 2015 & 2016	75-163
5	ALL INDIA AYUSH POST GRADUATE ENTRANCE TEST 2019	164-196
5	TEST YOUR KNOWLEDGE (MODERN ASPECT)	197-227
6	TEST YOUR KNOWLEDGE (UNANI ASPECT)	228-271

NIUM ENTRANCE EXAMINATION 2014

Q.1. Ghiza baad hammam may result in:
   A. Qai
   B. Suddae urooq
   C. Qarha shikam
   D. None

Q.2. which humma is caused by asbabe badiyah?
   A. Ghib
   B. Hummae yaum
   C. Shtrul ghib
   D. Aqtiqoos

Q.3 With which condition yarqan becomes radi (worse):
   A. Harrate jigar
   B. Salabat jigar
   C. Izame jigar
   D. Dared jigar

Q.4. which of the folloeing drug is recommended for treatment of hummae lasqa?
   A. Qurse afsanteen
   B. Matbookhe Aloo Bukhara
   C. Qurse Tabasheer
   D. None of above

Q.5 Illatuddajajah is synonym of
   A. Usre Tanaffus
   B. Khafqan

C. Zaheer
D. Wabaee Bukhar

Q.6 Which of the following is hummae lazimah?
A. Hummae istehsafiah
B. Hummae Kashafia
C. Hummae Lasqa
D. Hummae Tukhmia

Q.7 Which of the following is a type of sarsam?
A. Aqtiqoos
B. Maresmoos
C. Saqiroos
D. Nome of above

Q.8 Commonest cause of CVA is:
A. Arterial Thrombosis
B. Venous Thrombosis
C. Embolism
D. Tumour

Q.9 Reiter"s disease is characterized by:
A. Non specific Urethritis
B. Conjuctivitis
C. Reactive Arthristis
D. All of Above

Q.10 Epstein Barr virus causes all of the following except:
A. Infectious Mononucleosis
B. Measles
C. Nasopharyngeal Carcinoma

D. Burkitts Lymphoma

Q.11 A high amylase level in pleural fluid is suggestive of:
- A. Tuberclosis
- B. Malignancy
- C. Rheumatoid Arthritis
- D. Pulmonary Infaction

Q.12 A positive Romberg,s test is seen in:
- A. Disorder of posterior columns of spinal cord
- B. Unilateral labyrinthine dysfunction
- C. A& b both
- D. None of above

Q.13 Which of the following has longer shelf life?
- A. Samage arabi
- B. SAqmoonia
- C. Afyun
- D. Farfiyun

Q.14 Effect of Zarareeh on kidneys is an example of:
- A. Taseerae Bayeed
- B. Taseere Qareeb
- C. Taseere Awwali
- D. None of above

Q.15 What is common in Badle Qareeb,Badle Aqrab and Badle Bayeed?
- A. Ishtirake Taseer
- B. Ishtirake Jins

C. Ishtirake Nau
D. All of above

Q.16 which of the following drugs affect protein synthesis?
A. Chlorophenicol
B. Fusidic Acid
C. Aminoglycosides
D. All of above

Q.17 Solonum nigrum is botanical name of:
A. Kali mirch
B. Haleela Siyah
C. Mako
D. Amaltas

Q.18 Juze khas of mufarreh sheikhur rais is:
A. Daroonaj Aqrabi
B. Bifaij Fastaqi
C. Sumbuluteeb
D. Sandal Safed

Q.19 Acid Labile penicillin is:
A. Cloxacillin
B. Ampicillin
C. Phenoxymethyl Penicillin (penicillin 5)
D. Penicillin G (Benzyl Penicillin)

Q.20 Waraqul khayal is synonyms of:
A. Bhang
B. Dhatura
C. Afyun

D. Beesh

Q.21 Which of the following also known as Maddae Hayat?
   A. Majoon Najah
   B. Jawarish jalinoos
   C. Majoon Falasfa
   D. Majoon Murauwehul Arwah

Q.22 The term 'Drug' is derived from a...... word:
   A. Latin
   B. French
   C. Arabic
   D. Greek

Q.23 Berberis aristata DC is botanical source of:
   A. Zarishk
   B. Darhald
   C. Rasaut
   D. All of above

Q.24 Integredients of habbe shifa are:
   A. Tukhme Dhatura.Chob Chini.Zanjabeel.Samagh Arabi
   B. Tukhme Dhatura,Chob Zard,Zanjabeel,Samagh Arabi
   C. Tukhme Dhatura,Revend Chini,Zanjabeel,Samagh Arabi
   D. None of above

Q.25 Naura is used:
   A. To improve Face glow

B. To improve Eye sight
C. To strengthen and brighten the hair
D. To improve Hair

Q.26 .Molar concentration of isotonic fluid is:
A. 300 mosm/l
B. 350 mosm/l
C. 110 mosm/l
D. 0.9 mosm/l

Q.27 Which of the following is not found in circulating blood?
A. Fibrinogin
B. Prothrombin
C. Thrombin
D. Albumin

Q.28 which of the following statement is not correct?
A. Buffer system maintain acis base balance in the bady
B. Respiratory system and renal machenism play key role in maintaining body PH
C. Haemoglogin is one of the buffers that maintain acid base balance in the body
D. Erythrocytes have no role to play in maintaining PH of the body

Q.29 which of the following constituents is absent in serum but present in plasma?
A. Globulin

B. Fibrinogen

C. Albumin

D. iodide

Q.30 which of the following digestive juices does not contain any enzyme?

A. saliva

B. gastric juice

C. bile

D. pancreatic juice

Q.31 which of the following chemical agents is not a neurotransmitter?

A. Acetylcholine

B. Norepinephrine

C. Phenylalanine

D. Dopamine

Q.32 which nerves pass through the jugular foramen?

A. 9,10 and 11

B. 10,11 and 12

C. 8,9 and 10

D. 11 and 12

Q.33 the following structures lie in the posterior mediastinum except:

A. Vagus nerve

B. Phrenic nerve

C. Greater lesser splanchic nerves

D. Thoracic duct

Q.34 third part of duodenum lies in the:
   A. Transpyloric plane
   B. Subcostal plane
   C. Infrasternal angle
   D. Iliac fossa

Q.35 bifurcation of aorta is at the level:
   A. L 2
   B. L 2
   C. L 3
   D. L 4

Q.36 types of synovial joint are:
   A. 02
   B. 04
   C. 06
   D. 08

Q.37 kaboos is also known as:
   A. Zaghoot
   B. Jasoom
   C. Khaniq
   D. All of above

Q.38 nazla and zukam have similarity in:
   A. Maqame insebabe maddah
   B. Alamate kulli
   C. Mabdae maddah
   D. None of the above

Q.39 lahm,shahm,wa sameen are:

A. Aazae asliah
B. Aazae damwiah
C. Aazae raeesah
D. Aazae aaliah

Q.40 Ratubate ustuqussiya is also known as:
A. Ratubate jaunariya
B. Ratubate ghareeziyah
C. A & b both
D. None of the above

Q.41 Who is known as abul arwah?
A. Eropheloos
B. Jalinoos
C. Eraseestratus
D. Phrekides

Q.42 Which kind of balgham is har ratab?
A. Balghame maleh
B. Balghame hamiz
C. Balghame hulw
D. Balgham afis

Q.43 According to ibn rushd ,mauzoorate tibb are:
A. Sehte badan
B. Halite marz
C. Azaae mutashabehul wa murakkabah
D. Arkan

Q.44 According to ibn rushd akhlate arba are included in:
A. Azaae marakkabah

B. Azaae auwaliyah

C. Azaaee mutashabehul ajza

D. Azaae ghiziyah

Q.45 marze maddi is possible in association with:
A. Murakkab kaifiyat
B. Mufrad kaifyat
C. A & b both
D. None of theabove

Q.46 quwate ghaziaya is the name given to the following three quwa collectively:
A. Jaziba,hazma,dafia
B. Muhassila,mulassiqa,mushabiha
C. Masika,haima,dafia
D. Namia,tanasuliya,masika

Q.47 Caisson disease is due to:
A. Fat embolism
B. Thrombo embolism
C. Air embolism
D. Aminiotic fluid embolism

Q.48 Ghon focus is present in:
A. Progressive tuberculosis
B. Secondary tuberculosis
C. Milliary tuberculosis
D. Primary tuberculosis

Q.49 Female athlete triad consist of:
A. Amenorrhoea,disordered eating,osteoporosis
B. Hirsuitism,pcod,anxiety

C. Dysmenorrhoea,disordered eating,baldness

D. Infertility,disordered eating,loss of sleep

Q.50 Renal tuberculosis is infrred with which positive findings in urine examination:

A. Pus cell >10

B. Pus cell 10-20

C. Sterile pyuria

D. Few pus cell

Q.51 Most sensitive vaccine to heat is:

A. Measles

B. Typhoid

C. Polio

D. DPT

Q.52 Byssinosis is common in:

A. Textile industry

B. Sugarcane industry

C. Cement industry

D. Meay industry

Q.53 Grease coller is seen with:

A. Electrocution

B. Lightning

C. Thermal injury

D. Bullet entry

Q.54 Drawback of ozone as water disinfectant is:

A. Long time period for action

B. No viricidal effect

C. No residual germicidal effect

D. Teratogenicity

Q.55 Dry as a bone ,red as a beet ,blind as a bat,hot as a hare are the symptoms of:
  A. Opium poisoning
  B. Dhatura poisoning
  C. Aconite poisoning
  D. Ergot poisoning

Q.56 Marbling is the feature of:
  A. Mummification
  B. Purification
  C. Putrefaction
  D. Saponification

Q.57 The death from cyanide poisoning is due to:
  A. Anemic anoxia
  B. Anoxic anoxia
  C. Histotoxic anoxia
  D. Atagnant anoxia

Q.58 tareeqe laulabi is synonym of:
  A. Jal jantar
  B. Nadi jantar
  C. Grabh jantar
  D. None of the above

Q.59 Amale tabloor is equivalent to:
  A. Sublimation
  B. Crystallization
  C. Calcination
  D. Percolation

Q.60 Fine poweder of advia is known as:
- A. Selayah
- B. Malghamah
- C. Afshurdah
- D. Nughdah

Q.61 The book " Tafreehul Quloob" a translation by hakeem ahmadullah khan,is Persian translation of:
- A. Kital al- mukhtarat
- B. Risalah al-advia al qalbiah
- C. Mufarrehul quloob
- D. None of the above

Q.62 Nabze sagheer is characterized by:
- A. Harkate saree
- B. Harkate bate
- C. Kamie inqebaz wa imbesat
- D. Kamie sukoon

Q.63 Which organ is musharik of all organ?
- A. Jigar
- B. Qalb
- C. Dimagh
- D. None of the above

Q.64 Which of the following is not concerned with harkat wa sukoone nabz?
- A. Intezam wa adame intezam
- B. Ikhtelaf wa istawa

C. Khifiyate jirme shiryan
D. Miqdare imbesat

Q.65 the bual of patient of hasate kulliya is:
A. Ghaleez
B. Raqeeq
C. Siyah mayal
D. Sabzi mayal

Q.66 Post exposure prophylaxis is given in all except:
A. Rabies
B. Measles
C. Pertusis
D. Hepatitis B

Q.67 Which of the following is not true about jawarishe jalinoos?
A. Zafaran and mastagi are its ingredients
B. Mushk is one of its ingredients
C. Sumbullutib is one of its ingrediants
D. Khilanjan is one of its ingrediants

Q.68 Juze khaas of habbe siyah is:
A. Sammul far
B. Simab
C. Just
D. Afyun

Q.69 Which of the following books is not authored by akbar arzami?
A. Qarabadeene qadri

B. Risalah miqdariah
C. Mufarrehul quloob
D. Hudoodul amraz

Q.70 choose the correct pair from the following books and authers:
A. Dasturul atibba-abul qasim farishta
B. Ikhteyarate qatub shahi- mir mohammad momin
C. Zakheera nizam shahi – rustum jurjani
D. All of the above

Q.71 Bleeding from nipple is seen in:
A. Fibro adenoma
B. Duct ectasia
C. Duct papilloma
D. Abscess

Q.72 Peyronie' disease affects:
A. Breast
B. Vagina
C. Scrotum
D. Penis

Q.73 Which of the following is not the clinical features of the deep vien thrombosis?
A. Cell membranes
B. High grade level
C. Dilated superficial vien
D. Redness

Q.74 The most common site of rodent ulcer is:

A. Scrotum
B. Lower part of the face
C. Upper part of the face
D. All of the above

Q.75 Waldeyer's ring is situated around:
A. Nasopharyngeal tonsil
B. Pancial tonsil
C. Oropharyngeal inlet
D. Lingual tonsil

Q.76 In which stage of acute suppurative otitis media ,the ear drum show'Cart wheel appearance':
A. Catarrhat stage
B. stage of exudation
C. stage of suppuration
D. stage of complication

Q.77 The commonest cause of blindness with eys oain is:
A. cataract
B. glaucoma
C. conjectivitis
D. nano of the above

Q.78 Which of the following is called ,arze aa,?
A. Sue mizaj
B. Sue tarkeeb
C. Tafarruqe ittesal
D. None of the above

Q.79 Choose the correct sequence regarding sabab ,marz,and arz in hummae ufooni:
   A. Sabab- dared sar; marz –humma; arz –afoonat
   B. Sabab –humma ;marz- ufoonat ;arz – dared sar
   C. Sabab- ufoonat;marz humma;arz dared sar
   D. Sabab- ufoonat;marz-darde sar;arz humma

Q.80 Presence of habbul qara in the body is an example of
   A. Maraze maddi
   B. Maraze sue tarkeeb
   C. Maraze adad tabaee
   D. Maraze adad ghair tabaee

Q.81 Congenital absence of one finger of hand is an example of:
   A. Maraze waza
   B. Maraze mauza
   C. Maraze adad
   D. Maraze safaeh

Q.82 Tahajjure mafasil is related to:
   A. Amraze sue mizaj
   B. Amraze shakl
   C. Amraze majari
   D. Amraze waza

Q.83 Cardiac output is maintained at an elevated level:
   A. Throughout pregnancy
   B. In early pregnancy

C. In late pregnancy

D. None of the above

Q.84 Strawberry vagina is seen in infection by:

A. H.vaginali

B. T.vaginalis

C. C.albicans

D. H.simplex

Q.85 A plain x ray of the abdomen taken in the erect posture of a patient showed translucent shadow below the right side of the diagram.it indicates:

A. Gastric carcinoma

B. Peptic ulcer

C. Perforation of peptic ulcer

D. Gastritis

Q.86 The kussmaul's sign indicates:

A. Left heart failure

B. Mitral stenosis

C. Mitral regurgitation

D. Constrictive pericarditis

Q.87 Eczema ,pigmentation and ulcer over the lower part of leg indicate:

A. Arterial spasm

B. Buerger' disease

C. Acute venous obstruction

D. Chronic impairment of venous return

Q.88 In rokitansky – kuster – hauser syndrome:
   A. Vagina is absent
   B. Uterus is absent
   C. Ovaries & tubes are absent
   D. All of the above

Q.89 All are cause of urq ,except:
   A. Insdade fame rehm
   B. Ehtebase haiz
   C. Mailane rehm
   D. Warame unqur rehm

Q.90 Which part of the endometrium is shed during menstruation?
   A. Stratum compactum & spongiosum
   B. Stratum spongiosum & basalis
   C. Stratum basalis & compactum
   D. All of the above

Q.91 Fetal heamoglobin is:
   A. Alpha 2,gamma2
   B. Alpha 2,beta2
   C. Alpha 2,delta 2
   D. None of the above

Q.92 Fetal pulmonary maturity is assessed by:
   A. Bubble test
   B. Foam stability index
   C. Orange color cell
   D. All of the above

Q.93 The commonest cause of V V F in india is:
   A. Obstructed labour
   B. Pelvic surgery
   C. Radiotherapy
   D. Carcinoma of cervix

Q.94 Cause of kastre tams are all ,except:
   A. Riqqate dam
   B. Hiddate dam
   C. Ghizate dam
   D. Amraze jigar

Q.95 Association of nazla with sadaae har is an example of:
   A. Marze musallam
   B. Marz ghair musallam
   C. Marze batini
   D. Marze majaree

Q.96 Choose the correct pair form the following disease and organ:
   A. Shatra- anf
   B. Tarfa -chashm
   C. Bafa- qalb
   D. Aaqoona – dimagh

Q.97 Jiger is susceptible to:
   A. Amraze sue mizaj only
   B. Amraze sue tarkkeb only
   C. Amraze tafarruqe only
   D. All of the above

Q.98 Which of the following is not a kind of baule safed:
- A. Mukhati
- B. Fuqaee
- C. Ashqar
- D. Ahali

Q.99 The synonyms odf ziabeetus is:
- A. Barkaria
- B. Dolab
- C. Dawwarah
- D. All of the above

Q.100 Dawali is an example of:
- A. Amraze safaeh
- B. Amraze auwiya
- C. Amraze majari
- D. None of the above

Answer Key NIUM 2014

1.b, 2.b, 3.b, 4.a, 5.c, 6.c, 7.d, 8.a, 9.d, 10.b, 11.b, 12.c, 13.c, 14.a, 15.a, 16.d, 17.c, 18.a, 19.d, 20.a, 21.c, 22.b, 23.d, 24.c, 25.d, 26.a, 27.c, 28.d, 29.b, 30.c, 31.c, 32.a, 33.b, 34.b, 35.d, 36.c, 37.d, 38.c, 39.b, 40.c, 41.c, 42.c, 43.c, 44.c, 45. C, 46.b, 47.c, 48.d, 49.a, 50.c, 51.c, 52.a, 53.d, 54.c, 55.b, 56.c, 57.c, 58.b, 59.b, 60.a, 61.b, 62.c, 63.b, 64.c, 65.b, 66.c, 67.b, 68.d, 69.b, 70.d, 71.c, 72.d, 73.b, 74.c, 75.c, 76.a, 77.b, 78.c, 79.c, 80.d, 81.c, 82.d, 83.a, 84.b, 85.c, 86.d, 87.d, 88.d, 89.d, 90.a, 91.a, 92.d, 93.a, 94.c, 95.b, 96.b, 97.d, 98.c, 99.d, 100.c

NIUM 2015 Entrance Examination paper

1. **Which of the following may occur in imtela be hasbil quwa:**
   a. Infejare urooq
   b. Aiyae tamaddudi
   c. Ufoonate akhlat
   d. None of the above
2. **Gharoos is a:**
   a. Sala
   b. Khuraj
   c. Sartan
   d. Khanazeer
3. **According to ibn sina, harkate nabz is:**
   a. Harkate kammiah
   b. Harkate kaifiah
   c. Harkate wazaiah
   d. Harkate makaniah
4. **Which one of the following is not included in asbabe masika of nabz?**
   a. Qalb wa sharaeen
   b. Hajat
   c. Quwate haiwani
   d. Harkat wa sukoone badani
5. **Nabze azeem is mainly because of:**
   a. Shiddate hajate tarweeh
   b. Suqoote quwat

    c. Harkate qalb
    d. Miqdare khilt

6. **Zurqah and kumnah are disease of:**
    a. Uzn
    b. Anf
    c. Ain
    d. Asnan

7. **Morsarj is a disease of:**
    a. Lab
    b. Zaban
    c. Chashm
    d. Abru

8. **Ratq is associated with:**
    a. Male genital tract
    b. Female genital tract
    c. Respiratory tract
    d. Peritoneum

9. **Warame sulb is known as:**
    a. Shafaqaloos
    b. Saqiroos
    c. Farismoos
    d. Ilaoos

10. **Saudawl junoon is called:**
    a. Subara
    b. Mania
    c. Qutrub
    d. Hizyan

11. Phalen's sign is present in:
    a. Carpal tunnel syndrome
    b. Chronic nephritis
    c. Acute pancreatitis
    d. All of the above
12. The complication of hummae mevi is:
    a. Tassaqube amma
    b. Sarsam
    c. Zatur riya
    d. All of the above
13. Hummae yaum is caused by:
    a. Asbabe sabiqah
    b. Asbabe wasilah
    c. Asbabe badiah
    d. Asbabe qaimah
14. Sonukhas is:
    a. Safrawi
    b. Damwi
    c. Balghami
    d. Saudawi
15. Babinski reflex present during neurological examination of an adult patient Indicates:
    a. Peripheral neuropathy
    b. Upper motor neuron lesions
    c. Lower motor neuron lesions
    d. Autonomous neuropathy

16. Auther of moalajate buqratiah is:
    a. Abul hasan ali bin sehi rabban tabri
    b. Abul hasan ahmad bin Mohammad al tabri
    c. Ali ibn abbas majoosi
    d. Hunanin ibn ishaq
17. Choose the incorrect pair from the following:
    a. Baitul hikmat :abbasi period
    b. Ali geelani : mughal period
    c. Ikhtirate qutub shahi : mir momin
    d. Nizamuddin ahmad geelani : adil shahi period
18. Which of one the following books is known as " liber continens", in Europe:
    a. Jami-ul – mufradat
    b. Kitab Al –hawi
    c. Kitab Al –mukhtarat
    d. Kitab Al –shifa
19. Who included arwah in azae mufrada?
    a. Jalinoos
    b. Ismail jurjani
    c. Ibn rushd
    d. Allama sadeedi
20. There are how many types of juze amail of Tibb:
    a. 04
    b. 03

c. 02
d. 05
21. Maintenance of health is mainly associated with:
   a. Mizaj
   b. Asbabe arba
   c. Akhlat
   d. Quwa
22. Similax china linn. Is botanical name of:
   a. Chobchini
   b. Darchini
   c. Revandchini
   d. Kababchini
23. Muddate hayat depends upon
   a. Kammiate akhlat
   b. Kammiate ghiza
   c. Kaifiate quwa
   d. Mizaje qalbi
24. Which of the following is most har wa ratab?
   a. Lahme azli
   b. Arwah
   c. Khoon
   d. Lahme ghudadi
25. According to Unani tibb, taqaddum bil hifz is recommended in:
   a. Stationary good heaith

b. Declining good health
c. Old age
d. None of above

26. **The extent and pattern of distribution of drug depends on its:**
    a. Liqid solubility
    b. Difference in regions blood flow
    c. Extent of binding to plasma and tissue protein
    d. All of the above

27. **A khuraj having two or three openings is called:**
    a. Gharoos
    b. Saqiroos
    c. Shahdi
    d. Infialoos

28. **Weakness of which quwate jigar is responsible for istisqa:**
    a. Dafia
    b. Masika
    c. Mumaiyezah
    d. Hazima

29. **Mixing of water and sugar is example of:**
    a. Imtizaje sazaj
    b. Imtizaje haqeeqi
    c. Imtizaje har
    d. None of the above

30. The theory of 03 anasir was postulated by:
    a. Garohe mashaeen
    b. Ahle akseer
    c. Ashabe khaleet
    d. Buqrat
31. Tap –e muharreqa is a type of:
    a. Humma balghami
    b. Humma saudawi
    c. Humma safrawi
    d. Humma yaum
32. The synonym of husr is:
    a. Qabz
    b. Ehtabasul batn
    c. Imsakul batn
    d. All of the above
33. Warame kharateen is synonym of:
    a. Warme zaedae awar
    b. Warme amae sayam
    c. Warme amae diqaq
    d. Warme maae mustaqeem
34. Maddahe niqris is waste of:
    a. Hazme uzwi
    b. Hazme medi
    c. Hazme kabidi
    d. All of the above
35. Which is a type of basoore ghareeba:
    a. Zatul asi

b. Khafia zahira

c. Sheelam

d. All of the above

36. **Defferential diagnosis of sarsasme har should be made with:**

    a. Mania

    b. Malenkholia

    c. Shaqiqa

    d. None of the above

37. **The synonyms of uqal –e hawamll is:**

    a. Fawaq

    b. Uqal –e atfal

    c. Tashannuj –e nafaasi

    d. None of the above

38. **Which one of the following pairs is most sultable example of badale qareeb?**

    a. Suahaga madani :suhaga masnuee

    b. Suahaga madani :naushadar

    c. Suahaga madani :Raee

    d. Suahaga madani :jundbedaster

39. **Talteef is example of:**

    a. Taseere oola

    b. Taseere sanwiah

    c. Taseere salisah

    d. Taseere juziah

40. Mizaje saani tabaee of a drug is also known as:
   a. Zulkhassah
   b. Mizaje saani sannaee
   c. Murakkabul quwa
   d. None of the above

41. Mustajila is synonym of:
   a. Asgandh
   b. Aqar qarha
   c. Waj
   d. Bozidan

42. Glycoside calotropin is found in:
   a. Ushr
   b. Arnab
   c. Unnab
   d. Aqar qarha

43. If zanjabeel is added to turbud, the mushile balgham effect to turbud will:
   a. Increase
   b. Decrease
   c. Neither increase nor decrease
   d. Decrease after one hour

44. Jauahre munaqqa is obtained from:
   a. Raskapoor + Darchikna + sammul far
   b. Raskapoor + Darchikna + maveez munaqqa
   c. Raskapoor + Darchikna + Amla munaqqa

d. Raskapoor + shingraf + Amla munaqqa

45. Jawarish kamooni contains:
   a. Boorae Armani
   b. Gile multani
   c. Gile makhtoom
   d. All of the above

46. Plantago major linn. Is botanical name of:
   a. Lisanus saur
   b. Lisanul haml
   c. Lisanul asafeer
   d. Bazre qatoona

47. Makhrooj namooda means:
   a. Trituration of hajariyat till whole quantity of arq gets absorbed
   b. Mixing of dried powdered drug into liquid drug
   c. Grinding the drug and converting to paste
   d. None of the above

48. Covering of pills with saresh is known as:
   a. Ghilafe Hulami
   b. Ghilafe Qarni
   c. Ghilafe Duhni
   d. Ghilafe Shakari

49. Sheere amla is:
   a. Dried amla soaked in milk and dried
   b. Amla soaked in sugar and dried
   c. Extract of amla and mixed with milk

d. Fresh amla soaked in milk and dried
50. Which type of product forms when copper interacts with sirka khalis:
   a. Safeda kashghari
   b. Tutiya akhzar
   c. Sikanjbeen
   d. Zangar
51. Tukhm bedinjeer khotai is also known as:
   a. Kuchla
   b. Arand
   c. Jaml gota
   d. None of the above
52. Wormwood is English name of:
   a. Ood saleeb
   b. Afsanteen
   c. mazoo
   d. asrol
53. saqmunia is an ingredient of:
   a. Itrifal zamani
   b. Habbe banafsha
   c. Jawarishe shahrayaran
   d. All of these
54. Kussmaul's respiration was found on examination in a patient of renal failure. It indicates:
   a. Metabolic alkalosis
   b. Respiratory alkalosis

c. Metabolic acidosis
   d. Respiratory acidosis
55. **The differential diagnosis of raqaas should be made with:**
   a. Tassalube nukha mutadid
   b. Ikhtanaqur rahem
   c. Ikhtije mauroosi
   d. All of the above
56. **Exercise is a:**
   a. Voluntary movement
   b. Involuntary movement
   c. a & b both
   d. none of above
57. **Aims and objectives of Dalk are:**
   a. Strengthening of surgery
   b. Strengthening of the nerves
   c. Removing waste from skin
   d. All the above
58. **Hilton's law is a:**
   a. Procedure of surgery
   b. A procedure of reduction
   c. A rule of blood circulation in joints
   d. A rule of nerve innervations to the joints
59. **Saturday nights palsy is due to:**
   a. Injury to the axillary nerve
   b. Injury to the unlnar nerve
   c. Injury to musculocutaneous nerve

d. Injury to radial nerve
60. **Epithalamus is the part of:**
   a. Telencephalon
   b. diesencephalon
   c. mesencephalon
   d. metencephalon
61. **cell bodies of the upper motor neuron are located in the:**
   a. celebral cortex
   b. brain stem
   c. spinal cord
   d. outside the C N S
62. **rhomboid muscle shape is:**
   a. round
   b. oval
   c. trianglular
   d. diamond
63. **the following structure from the brain stem ,except:**
   a. pons
   b. medulla oblongata
   c. celebellum
   d. midbrain
64. **adrenaline and nor-adrenaline differ in their function:**
   a. in modifying respiration rate
   b. rate of oxygen consumption

c. effect of renal blood vassels
d. eosiniphil count

65. which of the following figures is correct in respect of specific gravity of whole blood?
   a. 1095 -1101
   b. 1028 -1032
   c. 1022 -1026
   d. 1052 -1062

66. Value of carbon dioxide (CO_2) tension of the cells during rest is:
   a. 40 mmHg
   b. 46 mmHg
   c. 20 mmHg
   d. 96 mmHg

67. Functional residual capacity includes:
   a. Expiratory reserve volume and residual volume
   b. Tidal volume and residual volume
   c. Expiratory reserve volume and inspiratory reserve volume
   d. Tidal volume ,inspiratory reserve volume and residual volume

68. Major phospholipid in pulmonary surfactant is:
   a. Triglycerides
   b. Phophatidyl glycerol
   c. Dipalmitoyphosphatidylcholine

d. Lipoprotein
69. Twelve by Twelve initiative is associated with:
   A. Anaemia
   B. Lodine deficiency
   C. Vitamine A deficiency
   D. All of the above
70. Which one of the following is not an example of tissue culture vaccine?
   a. PVRC Rabies Vaccine
   b. HDCV Rabies Vaccine
   c. PCECV Rabies Vaccine
   d. Dakar Yellow Fever Vaccine
71. Bangalore method of composting is also known as:
   a. Aerobic method
   b. Mechanical method
   c. Anaerobic method
   d. None of the above
72. In which of the following states, lathyrism is more common:
   a. Karnataka
   b. Maharashtra
   c. Madhya Pradesh
   d. Andhra Pradesh
73. Demographically, family size means:
   a. Total number of persons in a family

b. Total number of daughters born to a female
c. Total number of daughters that will be borne by a female as per prevailing mortality rate
d. Total number of children born by a female at a point in time

74. Joule burn is seen with:
   a. Electrocution
   b. Scalds
   c. Lightening
   d. Vitroilage

75. The vector of Japanese encephalitis in India is:
   a. Culex tritaeniorhynchus
   b. Culex vishnui
   c. Aedes aegypti
   d. Anopheles

76. The dilluent used for B.C.G vaccine is:
   a. Distilled water
   b. Normal Saline
   c. Dextrose Solution
   d. Ringer Lactate

77. Medullary Index of long bones helps to determine:
   a. Race
   b. Age
   c. Sex

d. All of these

78. The clinical diagnostic sign of hernia is:
    a. Compressibility
    b. Fluctuation
    c. Reducibility
    d. None of the above

79. The term von Recklinghausen's disease is used for:
    a. Generalized neurofibromatosis
    b. Generalized lipomatosis
    c. Localized neurofibromatosis
    d. None of the above

80. The term universal tumor applies to:
    a. Papilloma
    b. Lipoma
    c. Neurofibroma
    d. Haemangioma

81. The length of nasolacrimal duct is:
    a. 4 to 8 mm
    b. 8 to 12 mm
    c. 12 to 24 mm
    d. 24 to 32 mm

82. All the following are complication of sinusitis ,except:
    a. Mucocele
    b. Pyocele
    c. Meningocele

d. Meningitis
83. The goland's development begins between ----weeks of gestation:
   a. 8-10
   b. 5-6
   c. 3-4
   d. 7-8
84. XX chromosomes are required for:
   a. Testes development
   b. Ovarian development
   c. Fallopian tube development
   d. Uterine development
85. Sacrum is the denominator in:
   a. Breech presentation
   b. Face presentation
   c. Brow presentation
   d. Vertex presentation
86. Flow of menstrual blood into the fallopian tubes is called:
   a. Respective menstruation
   b. Remissive menstruation
   c. Retrograde menstruation
   d. Retrospective menstruation
87. Septic shock can be due to:
   a. Gram negative bacilli
   b. Gram positive bacilli
   c. Fungi

d. All of the above
88. Which is a DNA virus?
   a. Hepatitis A
   b. Hepatitis B
   c. Hepatitis C
   d. Hepatitis D
89. Myocraditis is most commonly caused by:
   a. Bacteria
   b. Fungus
   c. Virus
   d. Rickettsia
90. All are complication of chronic gastritis, except:
   a. Pernicious anemia
   b. Gastroesophagial reflux
   c. Peptic ulceration
   d. Gastric cancer
91. Apoptosis refers to:
   a. Uncoordinated cell death
   b. Cell death due to hypoxia
   c. Cell death due to radiation
   d. Coordinated and internally programmed cell death
92. The mechanism of fatty change in the liver in malnutrition is:
   a. Inhibition of fatty acid oxidation

b. Decrease in synthesis of lipid acceptor protein
c. Increase in synthesis of triglycerides
d. Alteration of mitochondrial function

93. Most commen tumor of appendix is:
    a. Carcinnoid
    b. Squamous cell
    c. Adenocarcinoma
    d. Argentaffin

94. Karyotype in turner's syndrome is:
    a. xO
    b. XXY
    c. XXX
    d. XXO

95. Which of these occurs only in uniovular twins?
    a. Foetus papyraceous
    b. Foetus compressus
    c. Foetus acardiacus
    d. Lithopaedion

96. Tobacco-pouch appearance is seen in case of:
    a. Genital tuberculosis
    b. Pulmonary tuberculosis
    c. Pott's spine
    d. Intestinal tuberculosis

97. Orf is caused by the virus that produces pustular dermatitis in:
   a. Sheep
   b. Reptiles
   c. Birds
   d. Humans
98. In Hippocratic teaching, to irrigate open infected wound which was used:
   a. Water
   b. Vinegar
   c. Milk
   d. None of the above
99. Components of each pair have some association, except one; choose one which is not correct:
   a. Penicillin: Howard walter florey
   b. Steven-johnson syndrome : adverse drug reaction
   c. Streptomycin: Gerhard Domagk
   d. Chloramphenicol :streptomyces venezuelae
100. Involvement of chest bone in Hadaba is termed as:
   a. Iltawa
   b. Reehul afrasa
   c. qa'as
   d. hadaba maqaddam

Answer Key NIUM 2015

1.c, 2.b, 3.c, 4.d, 5.a, 6.c, 7.c, 8.b, 9.b, 10.a, 11.a, 12.d, 13.c, 14.b, 15.b, 16.b, 17.d, 18.b, 19. C, 20.c, 21.b, 22.a, 23.c, 24.b, 25.b, 26.d, 27.c, 28.c, 29.a, 30.b, 31.c, 32.d, 33.a, 34.a, 35.d, 36.a, 37.c, 38.b, 39.b, 40.c, 41.d, 42.a, 43.a, 44.a, 45.a, 46.b, 47.b, 48.a, 49.a, 50.d, 51.c, 52.b, 53.d, 54.c, 55.d, 56.a, 57.d, 58.d, 59.d, 60.b, 61.a, 62.d, 63.c, 64.d, 65.d, 66.b, 67.a, 68.c, 69.a, 70.d, 71.c, 72.c, 73.d, 74.a, 75.a, 76.b, 77.c, 78.c, 79.a, 80.b, 81.c, 82.c, 83.b, 84.b, 85.a, 86.c, 87.d, 88.b, 89.c, 90.b, 91.d, 92.c, 93.a, 94.a, 95.c, 96.a, 97.a, 98.b, 99.c, 100.c

NIUM Entrance Examination 2016

1. **Which of the following can digest Carbohydrate, Protein and Lipid contents of diet?**
   a. Saliva
   b. Pancreatic juice
   c. Bile
   d. Gastric Juice

2. **Which of the following hormonal secretion is not regulated by the Pitutary Gland?**
   a. Thyroid hormones
   b. Adrenal Cortial hormones
   c. Ovraian hormones
   d. Pancreatic harmones

3. **Vital Capacity represants the sum of the following volumes:**
   a. Tidal volume, residual volume and inpiratory reserve volume
   b. Inspiratory reserve volume, expiratory reserve volume and tidal volume
   c. Tidal volume, residual volume and expiratory reserve volume
   d. Inspiratory reserve volume, expiratory reserve volume and residual volume

4. **Parathoromone (PTH) is secreted by the:**
   a. Oxyphil cells

b. Chief cells
   c. Parafollicular cells
   d. Follicular cells
5. **Which of the following nerves does not play any role in micturition?**
   a. Hypogastric nerve
   b. Vagus nerve
   c. Pudendal nerve
   d. Nervi erigentes
6. **Diencephalon is part of:**
   a. Mesencephalon
   b. Rhombencephlon
   c. Prosencephalon
   d. Telencephalon
7. **Which one of the following is a Telereceptor?**
   a. Hair cells in organ of Corti
   b. Krause end Bulb
   c. Meisner corpuscles
   d. Free nerve endings
8. **Mid portion of lung is:**
   a. Area of zero blood flow
   b. Area of intermittent blood flow
   c. Area of continuous blood flow
   d. Area of Trubulent blood flow
9. **Dynamic lung function is:**
   a. TV

b. PEF
c. ERV
d. Rv

10. **Bundle of his originates from:**
    a. SA node
    b. Av node
    c. Bundle branch
    d. Purkinji fibers

11. **Which one of the foiiowing is a branch brachiocephalic artery?**
    a. Left common carotid artery
    b. right internal carotid artery
    c. right commom carodit artery
    d. right external artery

12. **Floor of cubital fossa is mainly formed by:**
    a. medial border of brachialis
    b. pronator terries
    c. supinator
    d. anconeus

13. **Inguinal ligament is also called as:**
    a. ligament of cooper
    b. Ligament of poupart
    c. Ligament of Humphry
    d. None of the above

14. **Transverses thoracis originates from:**
    a. Anterior surface of lower sternum
    b. Posterior surface of lower sternum

c. Anterior surface of upper sternum
d. Posterior surface of upper sternum

15. **All the muscles of larynx are supplied by the recurrent laryngeal nerve ,except:**
    a. Cricothyroid
    b. Cricoarytenoid
    c. Transverse arytenoid
    d. Aryepiglotius

16. **Following cocci are gram-positive,except:**
    a. Streptococci
    b. Meningococci
    c. Pneumocaocci
    d. Staphylococci

17. **All are motile bacteria,except:**
    a. Vibrio
    b. Salmonella
    c. Shigella
    d. E.coli

18. **Choose the correct statement:**
    a. Excessive alcohol consumption is the most common cause fatty liver
    b. Reye's syndrome is also a cause of fatty liver
    c. Starvation may be cause of fatty liver
    d. All of the above

19. **Who is regarded as the father of cellular patholog?**
    a. William boyd

b. Rudolf Virchow
   c. John hunter
   d. William hunter
20. **Atrophy refers to:**
   a. Reduction of the number of parenchymal cells of an organ or its part
   b. Reduction of the size of the parenchymal cells of an organ or its part
   c. A and b both
   d. All of the above
21. **Sudden hypokalaemia is frequently seen in**
   a. Diuresis
   b. Diarrhoea from ulcerative colitis
   c. Diabetic coma
   d. All of the above
22. **Freiberg's disease affects:**
   a. Navicuiar
   b. Second metatarsal head
   c. Lunate
   d. Capitullum
23. **Which area is described as surgeon's grave yard?**
   a. Floor of mouth
   b. Tonsillolingual sulsus
   c. Diabetic coma
   d. All of the above

24. Adson 's test is positive in:
    a. Cervical rib
    b. Cervical spondylosis
    c. Cervical fracture
    d. Cervical dislocation
25. Buii's eye lamps provides an illumination of about:
    a. 200 candle power
    b. 300 candle power
    c. 400 candle power
    d. None of above
26. Internal use of penicillin G may be risky because:
    a. It may cause severe anaphylactic reaction
    b. It may cause severe organ toxicity
    c. It may indulge patients in reinforcement
    d. A &b both
27. Magnesium sulphate acts as drug mainly by its:
    a. Osmotic property
    b. Oxidizing property
    c. Chelating property
    d. Adsorption property
28. Paedriatic formation of aspirin are not allowed in countries due to the risk:
    a. Grey baby s yndrome
    b. Reye's syndrome

c. Rokitansky-kuster-hauser syndrome
d. a&b both

29. Which of the following is a prodrug?
   a. Dopamine
   b. Ampicilline
   c. Leodopa
   d. Prednisolone

30. Disease imported into a country, in which it does not otherwise occur, is called:
   a. Epornithikc disease
   b. Exotic disease
   c. Nosocomial disease
   d. Spodaric

31. Rigor mortis, First appears in:
   a. Heart
   b. Eyelids
   c. Fingers
   d. Muscles of law

32. Nuclear sexing is done by checking ....in cells:
   a. Nuclear Barr bodies
   b. Chromosome
   c. Genital organs
   d. None of the above

33. Which vitamin is also known as kidney hormone?
   a. Vitamin A

b. Vitamin B
c. Vitamin D
d. Vitamin K

34. Iceberg phenomenon of disease is related to:
    a. Laboratory
    b. Body
    c. Community
    d. Hospital

35. Health promotion is a component of:
    a. Primordial prevention
    b. Primary prevention
    c. Secondary prevention
    d. Tertiary prevention

36. For effective chlorination, desirable pH of water is :
    a. <7
    b. >9
    c. 7.2-7.6
    d. 8

37. Photometer measures all, except:
    a. Luminous flux
    b. Illumination
    c. Luminance
    d. Irradiance

38. Cyclic bleeding during first trimester 'is termed as:
   a. Welcome sign
   b. Implantation sign
   c. Placental sign
   d. Hegar sign
39. Robert's sign is present in:
   a. IVGR
   b. IUFD
   c. Abortion
   d. Pregnancy
40. Growth and development of the breast is called:
   a. Pubarche
   b. Adrenarche
   c. Thelarche
   d. Menarche
41. Complete absence of uterus when the......fail to develop:
   a. Wolffian ducts
   b. Mullerian ducts
   c. Fallopian tubes
   d. Ovaries
42. Commonest cause of secondary amenorrhoea is:
   a. Imperforated hymen
   b. T.B

c. PCOD
d. Prolactenaemia

43. Sub nuclear vacuolation indometrium is seen in:
    a. Menstrual phase
    b. Late secretary phase
    c. Early secretary phase
    d. Proliferative phase

44. Qib is related to:
    a. Jisme rahem
    b. Sadi
    c. Fame rahem
    d. Unuqurrahem

45. Choose the correct statement from the following?
    a. Bund kushad is related to men only
    b. Raqt is related to women only
    c. Aaqoona is related to men only
    d. A & B both

46. Author of "khulasatuttajarib" is:
    a. Mohammad akbar arzani
    b. Mohammad sharif khan
    c. Mohammad alwi khan
    d. Sahib abdul karim nagauri

47. Who is also known as galen of his time?
    a. Ibn sina
    b. Zakaria razi

c. Rabban tabri
   d. Abu sehel maseehi
48. **What type of phytoconstituents are found in drugs having mainly a'asir property?**
    a. Alkaloid
    b. Mucilage
    c. Tannin
    d. Resin
49. **Cassia fistula is:**
    a. Kali mirch
    b. Haleela siyah
    c. Mako
    d. Amaltas
50. **wasma is:**
    a. skin deseases
    b. a unani drugs
    c. an old surgery instruments
    d. a place in gold Greece
51. **the scientific name of nasoot is:**
    a. citrullus vulgaris
    b. ipomea turpethum
    c. pistacia lentiscus
    d. lactuca sativa
52. **seemab is about..........times heavier than water:**
    a. 13
    b. 18

c. 23
d. 28

53. **Pick out Correct Pair:**
    a. Tashkeen - - Taseere sani
    b. Idare baul - - Taseere Oola
    c. Talteef - - Taseere Sani
    d. Tajfeef - - Taseere Salisi

54. **Following colours are commonly used as the measure of Qeyas to assess the afficacy of drugs:**
    a. Red and Blue
    b. Blue and Black
    c. Black and White
    d. Red and Black

55. **Dawae Mutlaq acts by:**
    a. Madda
    b. Kaifiyat
    c. Surate nauiyah
    d. All if the above

56. **Which of the following is also known as Mizaje Sani Tabiee?**
    a. Zulkhassah
    b. Murakkabul Quwa
    c. Mutawfequl Quwa
    d. None of the above

57. **Which drug is Mufatteh:**
    a. Lateef and talkh

b. Lateef and Tursh
c. A & B Both
d. None of the above

58. Jauhare Rakapoor is Prepared by:
   a. Amale Taseer
   b. Amale Tabkheer
   c. Amale Taseed
   d. Amale Tajfeef

59. Ma'a-ul-Khilaf is also known as:
   a. Arq-e-Gulab
   b. Arq-e-Kevda
   c. Arq-e-Baid
   d. Arq-e-Kasni

60. Heera Kasees is usually prepared by:
   a. Iron & H2SO4
   b. Iron % HCI
   c. Iron & HNO3
   d. Iron & H2O

61. Very fine powder is obtained through:
   a. Sieve No. 40
   b. Sieve No. 60
   c. Sieve No. 80
   d. Sieve No. 120

62. Which of the following is chief ingredient of Barshasha?
   a. Ajwain Khurasani
   b. Dhatura

c. Afyun
d. Asrol

63. Amal-e-Tadkheen resembles the process of:
   a. Sublimation
   b. Distillation
   c. Sedimentation
   d. Decantation

64. Majoon Sarkhas is indicated mainly in:
   a. Deedane Ama
   b. Irqun Nasa
   c. Surate inzal
   d. Zeequn Nafas

65. In Roghan Haft Barg and Roghan Auraq:
   a. Ingredients of both are same
   b. Barg Bhangra is not included in Roghan Haft Barg
   c. Barg Madar is included is Roghan haft Barg, but not is Roghan Auraq
   d. Barg Dhatura is included in Roghan Auraq, but not in Roghan Haft Barg

66. Which of the following drugs is plant origin?
   a. Garde Sumaq
   b. Gaudanti
   c. Shakhe Gauzan
   d. Heera Kasees

67. Which One of the following is true about itrifal Ghudadi?
    a. It is used in Khanzeer
    b. Ghariqoon is one of its ingredients
    c. Mastagi is one of its ingredients
    d. All of the above

68. Choose the correct pair made from formulation and their main ingredients:
    a. Habbe Ahmar – Sammul Far
    b. Habbe Mulayin – Maghze Habbussalateen
    c. Habbe Mumsik – Afyun
    d. All of the Above

69. The Synonym of Illatuz – Zaib is:
    a. Quturb
    b. Mania
    c. Daul kalb
    d. None of the above

70. Bilateral Ptosis with resting divergence of the eye and lower facial weakness are feature of:
    a. Myasthenia gravis
    b. Parkinson's disease
    c. Wilson's Disease
    d. None of the above

71. Which of the following is not a cardinal feature of Leprosy?
    a. Anesthetic skin lesions

b. Thickened peripheral nerves

c. Pain

d. Acid - Fast bacilli on skin smears or biopsy

72. Burrow is an indication of:

a. Acne vulgaris

b. Herpes Labial is

c. Scabies

d. Herpes Zoster

73. Wood's light lamp is used to dignose:

a. Scabies

b. Ring worm

c. Eczema

d. None of the above

74. Infections mononucleosis is caused by:

a. Epstein barr virus

b. Betahemolytic streptococci

c. Gram positive bacilli

d. Coxsackei virus

75. Human is said to be muzmin when its duration is:

a. More than 21 days

b. Less than 14 days

c. More than 14 days but less than 21 days

d. None of the above

76. In humma, nuzj wa tahleel occur in:

a. Darjae ibteja

b. Darjae waqoof

c. Darjae tazaiyud
   d. Darjae inhetat
77. **For glycaemic control assessment, the best is:**
   a. GTT
   b. Fasting blood glucose level
   c. Glycated haemoglobin
   d. Fasting plasma glucose level
78. **Iritis commonly occurs in:**
   a. Grave's disease
   b. Rheumatoid arthritis
   c. Myasthenia gravis
   d. Addison,s disease
79. **Main characteristic of hypoglycemia is:**
   a. Rapid pulse
   b. Pyrexia
   c. Cold clammy skin
   d. Restlessness
80. **In human mutbeqa haqeeqi:**
   a. Blood is putrefied inside vessels
   b. Blood is putrefied outside vessels
   c. Blood is heated (josh wa ghalyan) without putrefaction
   d. All of the abov
81. **Important cause of illatuddajaj is:**
   a. Insibabe safra
   b. Insibabe balghame shor

c. Ihtibase riyah

d. All of the above

82. When nabze azeem, saree and mutawatir return toward normalcy:

   a. Firs tawatur disappears
   b. Firs surat disappears
   c. Firs lzm disappears
   d. All disappear simultaneously

83. Sabal is a disease of:

   a. Ear
   b. Nose
   c. Eye
   d. Teeth

84. Shatra, shirnaq and uqdah are related to:

   a. Eye lid
   b. Upper lip
   c. Septum of nose
   d. Pinna of ear

85. Chose the correct statement about Irqunnasa:

   a. It is so named, because it always affects women
   b. It affects a nerve known as Nasa in Unani medicine
   c. It causes excessive sweating in affected women
   d. All of the above

86. Asbabe lazima of pulse are all, except:
   a. Hawa
   b. Riyazat
   c. Makulaat
   d. Salabate shiryan

87. Mintaqa barida shumail lies:
   a. Between mintaqa shumali and mintaqa mautadila
   b. Between mintaqa shumali and khate istawa
   c. Between mintaqa mautadila shumali and qutbe shumali
   d. Between khate istawa and qutbe shumali

88. Which quwat is found only in humans?
   a. Quwate wahima
   b. Quwate samia
   c. Quwate Basira
   d. Quwate Natiqa

89. Ratubate ghareeziah is also known as:
   a. Ratubate urooq
   b. Ratubate tajaweef
   c. Ratubate ustuqussiyah
   d. All of the above

90. Aaraz are related to:
   a. Maddah
   b. Soorat
   c. Afaal
   d. Akhlat

91. Which of the following is hissi?
    a. Ilm
    b. Amal
    c. Tibb
    d. Fikr
92. Juzae ilmi of tibb deals with:
    a. Umoore tabiyah and asbab wa alamat
    b. Umoor tabiyah and ahwale badan
    c. Ahwale badan ,asbab wa alamat and tadabeera tahaffuz
    d. Umoor tabiyah ,asbab wa alamat and ahwale badan
93. Which of the following are asbabe faailli?
    a. Arkam wa mizaj
    b. Mizaj wa quwa
    c. Asbabe suttah zarooriyah
    d. Akhlat wa aaza
94. According to ashabe khaloot , yaksaniyte mizaj is:
    a. Haqeeqi
    b. Hissi
    c. Nauie
    d. None of the above
95. Mizaje motadil tibbi are of how many typees:
    a. 04
    b. 08

c. 09
d. 16

96. Mizaje motadil nauie bil qeyas iladdakhil is:
   a. Motadil haqeeqi
   b. Motadil tibbi
   c. Motadil hissi
   d. Ghair motadil tibbi

97. Which organ made of tarqeebe sani?
   a. chehra
   b. Chashm
   c. Raas
   d. All of the above

98. There are how many types of khoone ghair tabaee:
   a. 05
   b. 10
   c. 14
   d. 09

99. Balghame khan is abnormal in reference to:
   a. Zaiqa
   b. Qiwam
   c. Rang
   d. Boo

100. According to hukmae qadeem, qawat is:
   a. Kaifiyat
   b. Soorat
   c. A & b both
   d. None of the above

Answer Key NIUM 2016

1.b, 2.d, 3.b, 4.b, 5.b, 6.d,, 7.a, 8.b, 9.b, 10.b, 11.c, 12.c, 13.b, 14.b, 15.a, 16.b, 17.c, 18.d, 19.b, 20.c, 21.b, 22.b, 23.d, 24.a, 25.a, 26.a, 27.a, 28.b, 29.c, 30.b, 31.a, 32.a, 33.c, 34.c, 35.b, 36.c, 37.a, 38.c, 39.b, 40.c, 41.b, 42.c, 43.c, 44.c, 45.d, 46.c, 47.b, 48.c, 49.d, 50.b, 51.b, 52.a, 53.c, 54.c, 55.c, 56.b, 57.c, 58.c, 59.c, 60.a, 61.d, 62.c, 63.a, 64.a, 65.b, 66.a, 67.d, 68.d, 69.a, 70.a, 71.c, 72.c, 73.b, 74.a, 75.a, 76.d, 77.c, 78.b, 79.c, 80.a, 81.d, 82.a, 83.c, 84.a, 85.b, 86.d, 87.c, 88.d, 89.c, 90.c, 91.b, 92.d, 93.c, 94.b, 95.b, 96.b, 97.b, 98.c, 99.b, 100.b

AMU ENTRANCE EXAMINATION 2015 & 2016

1. Which of the following is prerenal cause of ARF (Acute renal failure)?
a. Glomerular Necrosis
b. Prostatic enlargement
c. Ureteric Stone
d. Heart Failure

2. Kashrat ehatlaam ma qabz '(nocturnal emission with constipation)ke liye mufid hai:
a. Bard sana e makki
b. Turbud
c. Roghan bed injeer
d. Isbgol

3. Qurs afsanteen mufid aor mujarrab hai:
a. Humma balghami ki Jumla aqsaam me
b. Judri me
c. Humma saudavi me
d. Humma dunj me

4. Zawi ul arwah dawa ki nishandehi Karen:
a. Roopa makhi
b. Shangarf
c. Usrab
d. Zahr muhrah

5. Sim mutalliq ka amal aor asar hota hai:
a. Kaifyat se

b. Kamiyaat se

c. Soorat e nooaiya se

d. Kamiyaat wa kaifiyat se

6. Amal Tajfeef ke baad gulab ke phool ke johar e lateef me kya farq padta hai?

a. Quwat talayeen badh jati hai

b. Talayeen kam ho jati hai

c. Quwat muhallila kam ho jati hai

d. Quwat muhallila badh jati hai

7. Habbe shifa me kon se ajzá shamil hai?

a. Joz Mashil, Magz badam, Magz bed injeer, zanjabeel

b. Suhaga, Ajwayin khurasani, Filfil siyah, Dhatoora

c. Shaham hanzal, usharah afsanteen, mastagi roomi, jozmashil

d. Joz mashil, revand chini, zanjabeel, samag arbi

8. Zaheer suddi me Habbe pechis ko kis dawa ke sath istimaal karte hai?

a. Roghan bed injeer ke sath

b. Roghan badam ke sath

c. Safoof mulayyin ke sath

d. Roghan ajeeb ke sath

9. Tiryaq arba ke taweel istemaal se kya muzrat hoti hai?

a. Dama paida ho jata hai

b. Qolinj ki shikayat ho jati hai

c. Qarha meda ho jata hai

d. Kuch nahi hota hai

10. Muhafiz janeen dawa ki nishadehi kijeye:

a. Darwanj aqrabi

b. Daar shishaan

c. Shadunj

d. Shaqaqil mishri

11. Sinus Tachycardia is usually due to:

a. Increase sympathetic activity

b. Exercise

c. Anxiety

d. All of the above

12. Potentially reversible cause of weight gain is:

a. Hypothyroidism

b. Familial obesity

c. Idiopathic obesity

d. None of the above

13. Kharooj muqad ki wajah hoti hai:

a. Astarkhai

b. Warmi

c. Morooshi

d. Warmi wa astarkhai

14. Bawaseer damia ke ilaj me mufeed hai:

a. Qurs kaharba

b. Habbe muquil

c. Majoon khabshul hadeed

d. All of the above

15. Malikhulya me istemaal kar sakte hai:
a. Ikseerein
b. Asanasiya
c. Anushdaroo
d. Tansheel

16. Leshar ghas ka cause hai:
a. Dam
b. Balgham
c. Sauda
d. Sauda wa safra

17. Suda damwi me kis rag ki fasd kholi jati hai:
a. Qeefaal
b. Safan
c. Akhal
d. Basaliq

18. Wajaul fawad ka mutradif hai:
a. Waja ul mafasil
b. Waja ul qatn
c. Waja fam meda
d. All of the above

19. Ushaba us dard ko kahte hai jo:
a. sar ke baalai hissa me hota hai
b. sar ke zeerein hissa me hota hai
c. poore sar me hota hai
d. Abroo wa bhaon me hota hai aor uske upper bhi

20. Khansi ke sath shokh surkh rang ka khoon kharij hota hai jab marz ka taluq hota hai:
a. Riya se
b. Mari wa meda se
c. Halaq se
d. Masoode se

21. Sala' naam hai us marz ka jisme:
a. Sar ke saare baal gir jate hai
b. Sar aor abroo ke baal gir jate hai
c. Sar ke agle hisse ke baal gir jate hai
d. Sar ke pichle hisse ke baal gir jate hai

22. Jo'ul kalb mei:
a. Khane ki khawahish had tabai se ziyada hoti hai
b. Khane ki khawahish khtm ho jati hai
c. Khane ki khawahish kam ho jati hai
d. None of the above

23. In palpation of abdomen "Guarding" indicates:
a. Generalized peritonitis
b. Localized peritonitis
c. Mild inflammation
d. Moderate inflammation

24. Galeez aor naqabil tahleel e riyah ke ijtimaa se paida ustushqa ko kahte hai:
a. Ushtushqa zaqi
b. Ushtushqa lahmi
c. Ushtushqa tabli
d. Ushtushqa amwi

25. Shiqafaloos ke ilaj me mufeed hai:
a. Gahre pachhne lagana
b. Halke pachhne lagana
c. Ghiza tark karna
d. none of the above

26. Dakhil urooq afoonat se humma ki kaunsi qism paida hoti hai:
a. Humma daira
b. Humma dayima
c. Humma yom
d. Humma diq

27. Taqllub al nafs kahte hai:
a. Derpa matli ko
b. Derpa tangi tanaffus ko
c. Derpa khafqan ko
d. Derpa khansi ko

28. Absent corneal reflex indicates:
a. Palsy of the ophthalmic branch of 5th cranial nerve
b. 7th nerve palsy
c. 2nd nerve palsy
d. a & b both

29. Shatrul ghab ki khilti bukharon ka murakkab hai:
a. Ghab wa naiba
b. Ghab wa mawaziba
c. Ghab wa lusqa
d. none of the above

30. Apex beat may not be palpable in the following case:
a. Emphysema
b. Pericardial effusion
c. Obesity
d. All

31. During history taking of a patient, it was found difficulty in swallowing with liquids and solids both. It indicates:
a. Achalasia of cardia
b. Oesophageal carcinoma
c. Laringeal carcinoma
d. Pharingeal carcinoma

32. Maadni dawa ko identify kijeye:
a. Argyreia speciosa
b. Hordeum vulgare
c. Conium maculatum
d. Lapis sanguine

33. Umron ke lihaz se darj zel advia ki muddat hayat ki sahi tarteeb kiya hogi?
a. Samagyat, barg, albaan, waitooaat, aor azharo faqa
b. Barg sagyaat, azharo faqa aor albaan wa tiyooaat
c. Albaan wa yatooaat, sagyaat, barg aor azhaaroo faqa
d. Barg, albaan wa tiyoaat, samagyaat aor azharoo faqa

34. Mahapat ki aanch den eke liye kitna bada gaddha khoda jata hai:

a. Ek feet mak'ab

b. Ek gaz makab

c. Barah feet makab

d. Kumhar ke anoe jaisa

35. Bees samai (poisonous) hota hai:

a. Insaan ke liye

b. Choohe ke liye

c. Dono ke liye

d. kisi ke liye nahi

36. Qurs Ghafis mufeed hai:

a. Poorane bukhar me

b. Nuqras me

c. Jiryan ud dam me

d. Sabat me

37. Mochras kis darakht se hasil kiya jata hai?

a. Keekar

b. Babool

c. Saimbhal

d. Naag phani

38. Sarwali ka konsa juz ghalba safra me mufeed hai:

a. Tukhm

b. Patte

c. Bekh

d. All of the above

39. Marookh kis dawa ko kahte hai:

a. Daant aor masoodon ke amraz me chaba kar istemaal karte hai

b. Maqam marz par malish ki jane wali roghani dawa

c. Maqam marz paar halke haath se mali jane wali dawa

d. Badan chidhak kar istimaal ki jane wali raqeeq khushbudaar dawa

40. Meetha zahar (sweet poison) hai:

a. Phosphorus

b. Aconite

c. Cynide

d. Indrayin

41. Shiqaq ul maqa'd ke ilaj me mufeed hai:

a. Marham safed

b. Qairooti

c. Aise paani me baithna jisme mazoo-gulnar – gul surkh, post anar ka joshanda ho

d. All of the above

42. Sarsaam ke kis qism ko Qarantis khalis kahte hai:

a. Sarsaam damwi

b. Sarsaam safrawi

c. Sarsaam balghami

d. Sarsaam saudawi

43. The causative organism of scarlet fever belongs to:
a. Virus
b. Bacteria
c. Protozoa
d. Fungus

44. **Agar suda jism me khoon ziyada hone lage to kis rag ki FASD kholi jati hai"**
a. Baasaliq
b. Akhal
c. Qifaal
d. Safan

45. **Sarsam balghami ka mutradif hai:**
a. Leshar ghas
b. Qarantis
c. Shifaqaloos
d. Hamrah

46. **Gurda reg ya ramal us waqt paida hota hai jab ke:**
a. Maddah zyada ghaleez aor leshdaar ho
b. Maddah ziyada ghaleez aor leshdaar na ho
c. Maddah miqdaar me kam ho
d. Maddah miqdar me ziyadah ho

47. **Acute renal failure is:**
a. Usually irreversible
b. Usually reversible
c. Usually gradual in onset

d. None of the above

48. Which of the following is not a sign of cardiovascular system?

a. Splinter haemorrhage

b. Tendon xanthomas

c. Xanthalesma

d. Spider navei

49. Buhran intiqali se murad hota hai:

a. Mariz ka inteqal kar jana

b. Marz ka dusri surat me muntaqil jo jana

c. Marz ka ksis bhi surat me muntaqil na hona

d. marz ka ek se dusre askhas me muntaqil hona

50. Which one water is beneficial for liver and spleen?

a. Ma'Shabia

b. Ma'Nahasia

c. Ma' Kaddu

d. All of the above

51. Kis mizaj ke askhas me azadi wa farakhadli ke sath istifrag ki ijazat di ja sakti hai?

a. Barid Yabis

b. Haar Yabis

c. Barid Ratab

d. Haar Ratab

52. Hijamat se anjam pata hai:

a. Istifrag sauda

b. Imala mawad

c. Dono

d. Koi nahi

53. Right coronary artery arises from which sinus?

a. Anterior aortic sinus

b. Right posterior aortic sinus

c. Left posterior aortic sinus

d. From anterior and posterior aortic sinuses

54. The plane passing through the body of lumbar 3 vertebra is:

a. Subcostal

b. Transpyloric

c. Transumblical

d. Intertubercular

55. Which of the following muscle is supplied axillary nerve:

a. Coracobrachialis

b. Teres minor

c. Teres major muscle

d. Bisceps brachi

56. The following muscles are supplied by the musculocutaneous nerve except:

a. Biceps brachii

b. Coracobrachialis

c. Triceps

d. Brachialis

57. The triceps muscle is supplied by:

a. Musculocutaneous nerve

b. Axillary nerve

c. Radial nerve

d. Median nerve

58. The glossopharyngeal nerve supplies the following:

a. Styloglossusus muscle

b. Stylopharyngeus muscle

c. Anterior 2/3 rd of tongue

d. Submandibular salivary gland

59. Foot drop is due to injury of:

a. Common peroneal nerve

b. Superficial peroneal nerve

c. Femoral nerve

d. Tibial nerve

60. Which of the following may be in normal variant:

a. R B B B

b. L B B B

c. Mobitz type II A.V block

d. None

61. Syndenham's chorea is present in:

a. Rheumatoid arthritis

b. Rheumatic fever

c. Encephalopathy

d. Cortical atrophy

62. The drug responsible for weight gain is:

a. Tricyclic anti-depressant

b. Corticosteroids

c. Sodium valproate

d. All of the above

63. Spleenomegaly indicates:

a. Portal hypertension

b. Right heart failure

c. Both

d. None

64. Pulsus paradoxus is present:

a. Pericardial temponade

b. Aortic regurgitation

c. Mitral regurgitation

d. All of the above

65. According to Ibn Sina normal color of urine is:

a. Baul e Utraji

b. Baul e Tibni

c. Baul e Zard

d. Baul e Abyaz

66. Daimi qabz me kya sahi hai?

a. Tez aor quwi mushilaat mamnou hai

b. Tez aor quwi mushilaat ki ijazat hai

c. Baqool wa fawaka muzir hai

d. Warzish ghair munasib hai

67. Da ur raqs marz hai:

a. Balghami

b. Saudawi

c. Damwi

d. Moroshi

68. Amal Khurm behatreen ilaj hai:

a. Nawaseer ka

b. Shiqaqul maq'ad ka

c. Bawaseer ka

d. Sabhi ka

69. Zosantaria me hota hai:

a. Ishal jisme khoon-peep ya ahma ki rutubatein kharij ho

b. Qabz jisme khoon ya peep kharij ho

c. Pechis se khooni ishal

d. None

70. Which is not the complication of Diverticular disease?

a. Abscess

b. Peritonitis

c. Haemorrhage

d. Stricture

71. Ek ASHA ka taqarrur darj zeil abadi par hota hai:

a. 2000 par ek

b. 20,000 par ek

c. 1000 par ek

d. 10,000 par ek

72. Ziyadatar qism ke ishal me zakhira tadiya (Reservior of infection) kon hota hai?

a. Insaan

b. Haiwan

c. Both

d. None

73. The most commonly employed chemical test to determine the presence of blood in stain:

a. Orthotolidine test

b. Benzidine test

c. Locard test

d. Horrock's test

74. Magnan's symptom is found in:

a. LSD poisoning

b. Chronic Dhatura poisonoing

c. Amphetamine poisoning

d. Chronic cocaine poisoning

75. Boiled egg is an example of:

a. Ghiza e lateef kasheer ul taghzia jaiyudul kaimoos

b. Ghiza e lateef Qaleel ul taghzia Raddiul kaimoos

c. Ghiza e kasheef kasheer ul taghzia jaidul kaimoos

d. Ghiza e kaseef Qaleel ul taghzia Raddiul kaimoos

76. "Corpus hippocratum" comprises of:

a. 72 volume

b. 82 volume

c. 92 volume

d. 62 volume

77. Revised national tuberculosis programme did not base on:

a. 70% sputum microscopy

b. 85% cure rate

c. Vaccination

d. DOTS

78. The size of "Respirable dust" is:

a. Less than 5 microns

b. Less than 10 microns but more than 5 microns

c. Upto 20 microns

d. Size does not matter

79. Ehatbaas ghair tabai ke asbaab me shamil nahi hai:

a. Quwat Dafiaa qawi ho jaye

b. Quwat masika qawi ho jaye

c. Quwat hazima zaeef ho jaye

d. Majari tang ho jaye

80. Konsa mosam bachon ke liye nihayat munasib aor mawafiq hota hai?

a. Mosam e rabia

b. Mosam e saif

c. Mosam e kharif

d. Mosam e sata

81. Kashtkari aor mazdoori ko kis qism ki riyazat me shamil karenge?

a. Riyazat A'ma

b. Riyazat Khasa

c. riyazat mutadil

d. Riyazat Arzia

82. Perfect Apagar score is;

a. 0-3

b. 9-10

c. 4-6

d. 10-12

83. RNA paramyxovirus is a virus of:

a. Small pox (Judri)

b. Measles (Khasra)

c. Mumps (Galsoo)

d. Influenza

84. HIV se mutasir afraad me ziyadatar afraad ko AIDS kitne din baad paida hota hai?

a. Daswein saal me

b. Daswein mah me

c. 5 we hafte me

d. 5 we din me

85. Which one is not a preventive regime in Dengue fever?

a. Control on mosquitoes

b. Vaccine

c. Isolation

d. All of the above

86. Yersinia pestis ke jarsoma ki khasiyat hai:

a. Motile (Musharik)

b. Koma ki shakl

c. Gram +ve

d. Gram -Ve

87. Ophitoxaemia means:
a. Chemical poisoning
b. Gaseous poisoning
c. Metalic poisoning
d. Snake poisoning

88. Dying deposition is recorded by:
a. Medical officer
b. Relative
c. Magistrate
d. Police

89. The ideal place to record temperature in dead body in from:
a. Rectum
b. Mouth
c. Axilla
d. Groin

90. Commonest source of epistaxis:
a. Roof of nasal cavity
b. Inferior turbinate
c. Middle turbinate
d. Anterior inferior part of nasal septum

91. Antrochonal polyn arise from:
a. Sphenoid sinus
b. Posterior ethmoid sinus
c. Ethmoidal sinus
d. Maxillary sinus

92. Hypovolemic shock is caused by:
a. A reduced circulating volume
b. Primary failure of the heart to pump blood to the tissues
c. A reduction in preload because of mechanical obstruction of cardiac filling
d. None of the above

93. Which one is true in case of healing by primary intetion:
a. Wound left open, heals by granulation contraction and epithelialisation
b. Wound edges opposed, normal healing and minimum scar
c. Wound initially left open, edges later opposed when healing conditions favourable
d. None of the above

94. In case of gas gangrene:
a. Causative organism is clostridium perfringens
b. Gas and smell are characteristics
c. Immuno compromised patients are most at risk
d. All of the above

95. Cushing syndrome is:
a. A diffused vascular goitre appearing at the same time as the hyperthyroidism
b. A simple nodular goitre, present for a long time before hyperthyroidism

c. A toxic nodule which may be part of the generalised nodularity

d. Hypersecretion of cortisol caused by endogenous production on excessive use of corticosteroids

96. Wondruff's plexus is:

a. Collection of blood vessels in the lateral wall of inferior meatus posteriorly

b. Collection of blood vessel around he middle turbinate

c. Collection of blood vessels in the little's area of nose

d. Collection of blood vessel over the roof of nasal cavity

97. Jacqemier's sign is also known as:

a. Chadwick's sign

b. Goodell's sign

c. Piskacek's sign

d. Palmer sign

98. Causes of primary post partum haemorrhage are except:

a. Atonic uterus

b. Retained uterus

c. Traumatic cause

d. Retained bits blood clots

99. Allane types of cervical biopsy except:

a. Punch

b. Wedge

c. Cryo

d. Cone

100. Age of elective surgical procedure for cleft lip is:

a. 1-1 ½ year

b. 1 year

c. 6 months

d. 6 – 12 weeks

101. Bandl's ring is synonym for:

a. Tonic uterine contraction and relaxation

b. Tonic uterine contraction and retraction

c. Irregular uterine contraction

d. None of the above

102. Drugs which can inhibit uterine contractions are:

a. Anticonvulsants

b. Tocolytics

c. Diuretics

d. Prostaglandins

103. Most common presentation Meckel's diverticulum:

a. Lower GI bleeding

b. Upper GI bleeding

c. Diarrhoea

d. Abdominal pain

104. Stone formation in gall bladder is enhanced by all except:
a. Clofibrate therapy
b. Ileal resection
c. Cholestyramine therapy
d. Vagal stimulation

105. All are complications of hydatid cyst in the liver except:
a. Jaundice
b. Suppuration
c. Cirrhosis
d. Rupture

106. Causes of bile duct strictures are following except:
a. Bile duct carcinoma
b. Acute pancreatitis
c. Trauma
d. CBD stone

107. Mamiran aor mamisha hai:
a. Maadni dawayein
b. Haiwani dawayein
c. Nabati dawayein
d. None of the above

108. Usharah revand hai:
a. Revandchini ka usharah
b. Darakht farfiran ka raaldar gond
c. Zaqum ka tarshah

d. None of the above

109. Agar kisi unani dawa ka asar rooh, akhlat, aor rutubat e shaniya tak ho to wo dawa:

a. Darja e dom ki hogi

b. Darja som ki hogi

c. Darja chaharum ki hogi

d. Mutadil hogi

110. Faad zahri aor tiryaqi dawayein:

a. Apne poore johar se dafa e zahar hoti hai

b. Bilkhasa apna fail anjam deti hai

c. Both are correct

d. None of above

111. Khubbazi ka nabati naam hai:

a. Malva Sylvestris

b. Althaea officinalis

c. Doronicum hookeri

d. Cordia Latifolia

112. Sharayit tajurba me nahi hai:

a. Tajurba insaan par kiya jaye

b. Dawa ko mukhtalif amraz me istemal kar liya jaye

c. Dawa ko mukhtalif miqdar me istimal kiya jaye

d. Dawa ke asrat daimi aor ibtadayi ho

113. Shukran ki samiyat ko door karta hai:

a. Roghan bilsan

b. Pujlusht

c. Jarjeer

d. Daarchini

114. Taghzia ke liye zaroori hai ki ghiza:

a. Balihaz miqdar wa kaifiyat zyada ho

b. Balihaz miqdar wa kaifiyat kam ho

c. Balihaz miqdar wa kaifiyat behtar wa munasib ho

d. None of the above

115. Mizaj Haar ko qayam rakhne ke liye kon cheez madadgaar sabit hogi:

a. Khooshi ki ziyadati

b. Mutwazan ghiza ki ziyadati

c. Kashrat wa riyazat ki ziyadati

d. All of the above

116. Munsif kis dimagi quwat ko kaha gaya hai:

a. Quwat mutkhayila

b. Quwat wahima

c. Quwat mutsarfa

d. His mustarik

117. Initial degradation of fatty acids in the mitochondria of cells is done by a process called:

a. Lipogenesis

b. Beta oxidation

c. Emulsification

d. All of the above

118. Which one is not vasoconstrictor agent?

a. Epinephrine

b. Augistensin II

c. Vasopressin

d. Bradykinin

119. Aaram ki halat me aorta me khoon bahne ki raftaar:
a. 3.3 cum/mt
b. 3.3 cum/sec
c. 33 cum/mt
d. 33 cum/sec

120. Kuryat hamra ki paidayish sabse pahle kis azoo se shuru hoti hai:
a. Yolk sal
c. Liver
c. Spleen
d. Bone marrow

121. Glomerular filtration rate ko kam karne wala awamil hai:
a. Dopamine
b. Platelets activating factor
c. CAMP
d. All of the above

122. Chronic paronychia is due to:
a. Candidiasis
b. Allergy
c. Bacterial only
d. Viral only

123. Pediculosis is due to:
a. Mites
b. Fungus
c. Lichen

d. Allergy

124. HLA-CW6 gene is associated with:

a. Psoriasis

b. Eczema

c. Keratoses

d. All of the above

125. Agar kisi mareez ke hathon ki ungliyon ke darmiyan degar maqamat par chhoti chhoti phunsiyan bahut kharish ke sath niklen aor ek shakhs se dusre ko ye marz phelne lage to iski mumkina taskhees ho sakti hai:

a. Basoor jawarsia

b. Basoor Safar

c. Jarb

d. Hikka

126. About the femoral nerve all statements are true except that:

a. It is the largest branch of lumbar plexus

b. It is formed by the anterior division of anterior primary rami of spinal nerve 1,2,3 & 4

c. It divides into anterior & posterior divisions

d. It lies in the femoral sheath

127. Which capacity of urinary bladder arises painful sensation for micturition?

a. 8 ounce (240 ml)

b. 4 ounce (120 ml)

c. 16 ounce (480 ml)

d. 32 ounce (960 ml)

128. The bone devoid of muscular attachment:
a. Cuboid
b. Talus
c. Navicular
d. Medial cuneiform

129. Darj zel me se kis me insulin receptor akhizah milta hai:
a. Hypothalamus
b. RBC
c. Renal tubules
d. Mucous membrane of intestine

130. Ushbi khuliya ke taluq se konsi baat durust hai:
a. Nissle granules me paye jate hai aor monosachride ki shakl me glucose ka istimaal karte hai
b. Nitrosome nahi paya jata hai aor galactose ki shakl me monosachride ka istimaal karta hai
c. Lysosome nahi paya jata aor fructose ki shakl me monosachrides
d. All of the above

131. Most of the synapses used for signal transmission in the central nervous system of human beings are:
a. Chemical synapses
b. Electrical synapses
c. Both

d. Nobe

132. Which of the following is not a gastro intestinal hormone:
a. Gastrin
b. Cholecystokinin
c. Trypsin
d. Secretin

133. Peptide hormone which causes sperm maturation in sertoli cells of testes is:
a. Oestrogen
b. Testosterone
c. FSH
d. LH

134. Quwat munfaila ka kaam hai:
a. Hayat bakhsna
b. Farhat bakhsna
c. Khushi aor gham ke ashrat ko qubool karna
d. All of the above

135. Chinese medicine ka nazariya YANG AND YIN kisne diya tha?
a. Fu Hsi
b. Shen Nung
c. Huwang
d. Hua Tu

136. Aza aslia woh aza hai jo:
a. Ghaleez khoon se bante hai
b. Ma-iyat khoon se bante hai

c. Mani se bante hai

d. Balgham se bante hai

137. Cules ka munjazb hokar kabid me jana:

a. Harkat kaifiya hai

b. Harkat kamiya hai

c. Harkat makaniya hai

d. Harkat ainiya hai

138. Safra kurrasi:

a. Safra bilzat khud jal jata hai

b. Jala hua sauda shamil ho jaye

c. Jala hua balgham shamil ho jaye

d. Ghaleez balgham shamil ho jaye

139. Jalinoos ne balgham ke namkeen hone ki wajah se kisko qarar di hai:

a. Hararat

b. Burudat

c. Ahtraq

d. Ufunat

140. Kitab Firdausul hikmat ka musannif hai:

a. Tabri

b. Majoosi

c. Sina

d. Maseehi

141. Darj zel me konsi kitab buqrat ki nahi hai:

a. Kitabul ajna

b. Kitab tabiyatul insaan

c. Kitabul akhlat

d. Moalijat buqratia

142. Qadeem unaniyon ka tabbe aowal tha:

a. Asqali bus awal

b. Amhotib

c. Buqrat

d. Jalinoos

143. Hazm medwi wa hamumi:

a. Alag alag hai

b. Ek he hai

c. Dono sahi hai

d. Koi nahi

144. Hikka me mufid hai:

a. Roghan Qust se dalk armaul jabn se tarteeb

b. Roghan qust se dalk aor maul lahm se tarteeb

c. Roghan gul se dalk aor maul lahm se tarteeb

d. Roghan gul se dalk aor maul jabn se tarteeb

145. Generalised pruritus, pigmentation, spider naevi and palmer erythema can be caused by:

a. Involvement of kidney

b. Impetigo

c. Involvement of liver

d. Sclerosis

146. The deficiency of zinc is related with:

a. Acrodermatitis enteropathica

b. Phrynoderma

c. Angular stomatitis

d. All of the above

147. Balano-posthisis is due to:

a. Candidiasis

b. Deficiency of biotin

c. Excess of mineral intake

d. None of the above

148. Jun ek khas qism jo jildi mslimat se chaspa aor iske ander ghusi rahti hai, shanakht kijeye:

a. Qaml

b. Shiban

c. Qamqaam

d. Iltul na'ma

149. Balon ke girne ke sabab ki shinakht kijeye:

a. Qilat ghiza wa takhlakhul jild

b. Yaboosat, rutubat, fasid mawad

c. Sa'fa, quruh, iltul naám

d. all of the above

150. Triple test kya detect karne ke liye kiya jata hai?

a. Stein Leventhal syndrome

b. Down's syndrome

c. Turner's syndrome

d. Hydrocephalus

151. Polyhydramnios ka complication nahi hai:

a. Eclampsia

b. Preeclampsia

c. Malpresentation

d. Pre term labour

152. Abnormal placenta ki woh kaunsi qism hai jisme chord membrane se judi hoti hai:
a. Placenta succenturiata
b. Placenta extrachorialis
c. Battle dove placenta
d. Velamentous placenta

153. Colostrum ka juz nahi hai:
a. Protein
b. Vitamin B
c. Fat
d. Potassium

154. Nazariya aqleem ka mojid kise samja jata hai:
a. Hasparkas
b. Hebagoras
c. Batlimoos
d. Ibn Sina

155. Elevated A.S.O. titer is found in:
a. Infection of Salmonella typhi
b. Infection of Corynebacterium diphtheria
c. Infection of Staphylococcus aureus
d. Infection of Streptococcus pyogenes

156. Which kidney stone is not radio opaque?
a. Pure uric acid stone
b. Phosphate stone
c. Oxalate stone
d. b & c

157. The stomach wall is found to be thick & leathery in cases of poisoning due to:
a. Organophosphorus
b. Lead
c. Copper sulphate
d. Carbolic acid

158. Most common site of carcinoma of stomach is:
a. Body of stomach
b. Fundus of stomach
c. Antrum of stomach
d. Cardia of stomach

159. High incidence of carcinoma of stomach is associated with blood group:
a. A
b. B
c. AB
d. O

160. Warm haar ke kis darje me warm me ziyadati hoti hai aor iska huzm bhi badhne lagta hai:
a. Darja e intiha
b. Darja ibtida
c. Darja Tazyid
d. Darja inhitat

161. Erythropoietin is produced by:
a. Liver
b. Lungs

c. Bone marrow

d. Kidney

162. Saudawi basoor ki missal hai:

a. Masameer

b. Nafataat

c. Shaleel

d. Jawarsia

163. Qurs banane ke liye jis rabita ka aksar istimal karte hai woh hai:

a. Samag arbi

b. Jalatain

c. Shahad

d. Glycerin

164. Basra basta lafz mustamil hai:

a. Tukhm kitan ko

b. Tukhm kasoos ko

c. Tukhm kasini ko

d. Tukhm kakanj ko

165. Zer pastan hijamat bil shurt kis marz me karte hai?

a. Ehatbaas-tams me

b. Kashrat -tams me

c. Usr-tams me

d. Uqar

**166. Jis kisi dawa ko jalakar us ka dukhan (dhunwa) jo hawa ya gas ki shakl me hota hai-usko khas tarkeeb ke zariye kisi khas maqam tak pahunchaya jata hai –us amal ko tibbi istilah me kaha jata hai:

a. Inkibab
b. Bukhoor
c. Zarooq
d. Nushooq

167. Aqsaam ghiza ki rooh se reshedaar, luaabdaar sabziyan, sukha gosht, charbiyan, mukhtalif qism ki daalein maslan chana, matar, urd baqla wagairah kis qism ki ghiza se taluq rakhti hai:

a. Ghiza lateef kaseer ul taghzia
b. Ghiza lateef Qaleelul taghzia
c. Ghiza kaseef kaseer ul taghzia
d. Ghiza kaseef Qaleel ul taghzia

168. Hamam ka paani jism me konsi kaifiyat paida karta hai:

a. Hararat
b. Burudat
c. Koi nahi
d. both a &b

169. Ghiza me pahunchne ke baad tabdeel ho jaye lekin juz badan hone ki salahiyat na rakhti ho:

a. Ghiza mutaliq
b. Dawa mutadil
c. Dawa mutaliq
d. Dawa simmi

170. Mamnuaat qai ki nishandehi Karen:

a. Mufrat farbahi

b. Sara'

c. Falij

d. Sojish hanjrah

171. Amal hijamat se qbl mariz ko kya dena munasib hoga?

a. Sharbat faulad

b. Sharbat deenar

c. Sharbat Anar

d. Sharbat sandal

172. Cavernous sinus contains of the following except:

a. Optic nerve

b. Internal carotid artery

c. Oculomotor nerve

d. Trigeminal nerve

173. The shortest extraocular muscle is:

a. Superior oblique

b. Inferior oblique

c. Superior rectus

d. Inferior rectus

174. Most uncommon type of latent squint is:

a. Esophoria

b. Exophoria

c. Hyperphoria

d. Cyclophoria

175. Anterior segment of the eye ball includes structures lying in front of the:
a. Iris
b. Crystalline lens
c. Vitreous body
d. Cornea

176. The best drug for treating bradycardia is:
a. Atropine
b. Glycopyrrolate
c. Scopolamine
d. Ipratropium

177. Short acting local anaesthetic is:
a. Bupivacaine
b. Mepivacaine
c. Ropivacaine
d. Lidocaine

178. The best inhalation anaesthetic for induction in children is:
a. Isoflurane
b. Deflusane
c. Nitrous oxide
d. Sevoflurane

179. Reactionary haemorrhage ki wajah nahi hai:
a. Slipping of ligature
b. Dislodgement of blood clot
c. Hypotension
d. Hypertension

180. Strangulation kis hernia me ziyada paya jata hai:

a. Indirect inguinal hernia

b. Incisional hernia

c. Umblical hernia

d. Femoral hernia

181. Superior rectal artery is a continuation of:

a. Superior mesenteric artery

b. Internal iliac artery

c. Inferior mesenteric artery

d. Internal pudendal artery

182. Warm haar ke awamil me darj zel konsi dawa istimaal ki jati hai?

a. Muhallilat

b. Markhyat

c. Rawada'

d. All of the above

183. Darj-zel me konsi dawa mughalliz mani hai?

a. Samandar sokh

b. Samaq

c. both

d. None

184. Maúl bazr taiyar hota hai:

a. Bazariya joshanda

b. Bazariya khisanda

c. Bazriya takhmeer

d. Bazariya ta'riq

185. Konsi dawa munfi't nahi hai:
a. Sher madar
b. Biladar
c. Zangar
d. Zararih

186. Gharah kis azu ke marz me istimaal kiya jata hai?
a. Aankh
b. Naak
c. Kaan
d. Halq

187. Tribulus terrestris kis dawa ka nabati naam hai?
a. Hanzal
b. Chaksu
c. Khar khusk
d. None of the above

188. Liquiritin paya jata hai:
a. Suddab
b. Karfas
c. Asl alsoos
d. Kabab chini

189. Itrifal me haleela jaat ki teeno qismo ka istemaal karte hai:
a. Tanqia ke liye
b. Taqwiyat ke liye
c. Both

d. None

190. Murakkab advia me teen guna shahad shamil ki jati hai:

a. Murakkab ke tahaffuz ke liye

b. Murakkab ka maza durust karne ke liye

c. Murakkab me hararat aor latafat paida karne ke liye

d. All of the above

191. Jalmandrah hai:

a. Ek qism ki dawa

b. Ek bartan jot el nikaalne me kaam aata hai

c. Ek qism ka masala jo jodne ke kaam aata hai

d. Aanch dene ka ek tareeqa jo kushta banane me kaam aata hai

192. HIV infects and destroyes:

a. CD-8 cells

b. CD-4 cells

c. CD-1 cells

d. CD-12 cells

193. Alaamat e joharia woh alaamat hai:

a. Jo mizaj ke ehtadal ko zahir karti hai

b. Jin ka taluq aza ke afaal se hota hai

c. Jin ke zariye badan ki shakht ki durustagi wa udam durustagi ka pata chalta hai

d. None of the above

194. Laung ke hamrah kharl karne par siyah rang hota hai:

a. Kushta tamba

b. Kushta abrak safed

c. Kushta abrak siyah

d. Kushta nuqra

195. Kisi dawa ke ajza lateefa utriya hasil karne ke liye konsa aala istimaal karte hai?

a. Qara ambeq

b. Tariq hubli

c. Nal bhabka

d. Hamam ma'iya

196. Hamam nariya ke mutaliq sahi hai:

a. Hamam ma'iya bhi kahte hai

b. Deg par deg bhi kahte hai

c. Qara ambeq ki ek qism hai

d. All of the above

197. Distillation apparatus kahte hai:

a. Tariq zujaji

b. Tariq hubli

c. Teju jantar

d. Tariq lolbi

198. Tila kaseed kiya jata hai:

a. Qara ambeq se

b. Deg bhabka se

c. Patal jantar se

d. Distillation plant se

199. Kushta go'danti banane ke liye paahle isko kharl karte hai:

a. Arq gulab me

b. Aab tarbooz me

c. Aab anar me

d. Aab gheegawar me

200. Dahanaab ka mal kiya jata hai:

a. Abrak safed par

b. Abrak siyah par

c. Dono par

d. Kushta banane ke liya

201. Zawiulnufoos kahte hai:

a. Woh asya jo zawiul ajsad aor zawi ul arwah me rabita ka kaam kare

b. Maslan fitkari, shora noshadar

c. Both

d. None of the above

202. Neuroblastoma ki sab se common site konsi hai:

a. Paravertebral retroperitoneum

b. Posterior mediastinum

c. Pelvis

d. Adrenal gland

203. 10 yrs tak ke bachon me iodine ki daily requirement hai:

a. 40-120 microgram

b. 120-180 microgram

c. 180-200 microgram

d. 200 -240 microgram

204. Dysmenorrhoea kis me aam hota hai?
a. Uterus septus
b. Uterus unicornis
c. Bicornuate uterus
d. Hypoplastic uterus

205. Hormone replacement therapy kis hormone ki kami ko poora karne ke liye dijati hai:
a. LH
b. FSH
c. Progesterone
d. Oestrogen

206. Nabothian follicles kis marz ke characteristic feature hai?
a. Acute endometritis
b. Chronic endometritis
c. Acute cervicitis
d. Chronic cervicitis

207. Pregnancy is a state of:
a. Respiratory acidosis
b. Respiratory alkalosis
c. Both may be present
d. None of the above

208. Eclampsia ke daure ziyadatar kab padne shuru hote hai?
a. Intrapartum
b. Antepartum
c. Intercurrent

d. Postpartum

209. Maximum no. of oogenia found in female gonads at the age of:
a. 16 wks of pregnancy
b. Puberty
c. 20 wks of pregnancy
d. At birth

210. Ovulation occurs soon after the formation of:
a. Primary oocyte
b. After puberty
c. Secondary oocyte
d. Before menopause

211. Common causes of first trimester abortion are except:
a. Genetic factor
b. Luteal phase defect
c. Cervico uterine factor
d. Deficient progesterone

212. Ushtushqa dimag ka shuba hota hai agar head circumference badhta hai:
a. 3 cm/mth se ziyada
b. 2 cm/mth se ziyada
c. 1 cm/mth se ziyada
d. 4 cm/mth se ziyada

213. Amraz atfal me kis age tak ke bachae aate hai:
a. 10 yrs se kam
b. 12 yrs se kam

c. 14 yrs se kam

d. 18 yrs se kam

214. Ek saal ke bache ki qalb ki raftaar hoti hai:

a. 110 beats/min

b. 100 beats/min

c. 140 beats/min

d. 120 beats/min

215. Kuzaz khalqi me mariz ka sar jhuk jata hai:

a. Peeche ki taraf

b. Aage ki taraf

c. Kisi ek janib

d. Sidha rahta hai

216. Pickup correct one:

a. Uterus develops from mullerian ducts (paramesonepheric ducts)

b. Isthmus is a constricted region in the lower part of the uterus, which forms the lower uterine segment at full term of pregnancy

c. Most fixed part of the uterus is supra vaginal cervix

d. All are correct

217. A fully mature corpus luteum measures about:

a. 18-20 microns

b. 100 microns

c. 150 microns

d. 18-20 mm

218. Following are the high risk group for cervical cancer except:
a. 25-30 yrs of age
b, Multi parity
c. Multiple sexual partner
d. Infertile woman (Uqr)

219. The commonest cause of menorrhagia in child bearing age is:
a. Fibroid
b. Endometrial carcinoma
c. Pelvic endometriosis
d. Adenomyosis

220. Incubation period of typhoid fever:
a. 1-4 daays
b. 1-4 weeks
c. 10-14 days
d. 10-14 weeks

221. Hindustan me sabse pahle census kis saal hui thi?
a. 1871
b. 1881
c. 1971
d. 1981

222. W.H.O ki air pollution se mutaliq laboratory Hindustan me kahan hai?
a. Delhi
b. Calcutta

c. Chennai

d. Nagpur

223. Sabaat ka sabab hai:

a. Burudat ka ghlaba

b. Rutubat ka ghalba

c. Badan me khoon ki kasrat

d. All of the above

224. Faras ul baul me mufeed hai:

a. Gukqand usli

b. Maúl usl

c. Ma;us shair

d. Maúl jabn

225. Istafrag se pahle Nuzj:

a. Zaroori hai

b. Ghair zaroori hai

c. Sirf ghalba safra me ghair zaroori hai

d. Nuzj ke bagair baaz surton me wajib hai

226. Amraz bah me mareezon ke liye qabz ki behatreen dawa hai:

a. Sana maki

b. Turbud

c. Saqmoonia

d. Ispgol musallim

227. Dawa al moz mustamil hai:

a. Zaturriya me

b. Zatul janb me

c. Shahiqa me

d. Shaqeeqa me

228. Qalbi ghasi ka sabab hota hai:

a. Qalb ka warm haar

b. Qalb ka imtila

c. Qalb ka warm muzmin

d. Qalb ka suddah

229. Development of Q waves in ECG suggestive of:

a. Angina pectoris

b. Ventricular fibrillation

c. Atrial fibrillation

d. Myocardial infarction

230. Which of the following causes mouth ulcer?

a. Candidiasis

b. Measles

c. Behcet's disease

d. All of the above

231. Istishqa ka aam sabab hota hai:

a. Hazm me'wi ka zoaf

b. Hazm me'di ka zoaf

c. Hazm kabdi ka zoaf

d. All of the above

232. Riya ke qarha ko kahte hai:

a. Sil

b. Zatur riya

c. Diq

d. None of the above

233. Dawali kahte hai:

a. Dorane sar ko

b. Pindli aor qadam rag ke phail jane ko

c. Khusia ke rag ke phail jane ko

d. Jigar ki rag ke phail jane ko

234. Ashab khaleet ke nazariya ke mutabiq anasir ki tadad:

a. 3

b. 4

c. 5

d. Anaseer kashirah

235. Aza basita ka mizaj:

a. Bil arz

b. Bilzaat

c. dono

d. koi nahi

236. Darj zel me sabse ziyada har azu konsa hai:

a. Qalb

b. Jigar

c. Laham

d. Shaham

237. Balgham jassi hai:

a. Raqeeq balgham

b. Pighli hui kaanch ki tarah

c. Nihayat ghaleez balgham

d. Pheeka balgham

238. Quwat mustarjá konsi quwat hai:

a. Quwat mutkhaiyala

b. Quwat fai'la

c. Quwat munfaila

d. Quwat hafiza

239. Ghisa a'm raqeeqa kahan pai jati hai:

a. Ma al bain

b. Dimag

c. Raham

d. Riya

240. Dorane khoon rewi ka ka mojid kon hai?

a. Qarshi

b. Ibn sina

c. Jalinoos

d. Allama Nafees

241. Azu damwi hai:

a. Urooq

b. Laham

c. Aasáb

d. Vatr

242. Jundi shapoor kiya tha?

a. Ek badshah

b. Ek tabeeb

c. Tibbi madarsa

d. Tibbi kitab

243. Hindi tibb mei qadeem tareen tabeeb kisko mana jata hai?
a. Chark
b. Sushrat
c. Wagbhatt
d. Naag arjun

244. Psoas test done for the diagnosis of:
a. Cholecystitis
b. Cholidocolithiasis
c. Acute pancreatitis
d. Retrocaecal appendicitis

245. Meckel's diverticulum arises from:
a. Hind gut
b. Foregut
c. Mid gut
d. All of the above

246. Disposal of waste ke tareeqon me composting ke darj zel naamo me konsa naam baqi teeno se mukhtalif hai:
a. Banglore method
b. Hot fermentation method
c. Anaerobic method
d. Mechanical composting

247. Phossy jaw paya jata hai:
a. Sammulfar ki simiyat me
b. Iodine ki simmiyat me
c. Phosphorus ki simmiyat me

d. Para ki simmiyat me

248. Namkeen pani me doobne se maut amooman kitne der me hoti hai?

a. 4-5 minute

b. 8-12 minutes

c. 8-10 minutes

d. 5-30 minutes

249. Nisha angasht kahte hai:

a. Dactylography

b. Dermatoglypics

c. Galton system

d. All

250. I.P.C means for:

a. International patent code

b. Indian penal code

c. Indian patent code

d. None

251. Hindustan me naásh barari (exhumation) kitni muddat tak ki jasakti hai:

a. 5 yrs

b. 2 yrs

c. 7 yrs

d. No limitation

252. Byan nazeeí (dying declaration) ho sakta hai:

a. Magistrate

b. Wakeel

c. Police officer

d. Samaj ka koi muazziz shakhs

253. A BMI of 26 is indicative of:

a. Moderate obesity

b. Pre obese

c. Under weight

d. Normal weight

254. In a 70 kg adult male, the volume (in liter) of total body water is:

a. 42 L

b. 32 L

c. 14 L

d. 28 L

255. Harkat badni se wa harkat nafsani se jism ki tahleel hoti hai:

a. Arkan ki

b. Akhlat ki

c. Aza'ki

d. Quwat ki

256. Cheyne stroke breathing is found in all except:

a. Anxiety

b. Ventricular failure

c. Cerebrovascular accident of brain

d. Sleep

257. Which is not a defect of image formation:

a. Hyperopia

b. Myopia

c. Emmetropia

d. Presbyopia

258. Ek qism ki khusunat jo jild me paida hoti hai, iska rang siyahi ma'il aor gahe surkhi ma'il hota hai:

a. Nibatul lail

b. Jarb ratab

c. Humeqah

d. Qoba

259. Baalon ko daraz karne wali dawa:

a. Choona

b. Hadtal

c. Bakai'n

d. Fitkari

260. Konsa wart painful hota hai:

a. Common wart

b. Genital wart

c. Plane wart

d. Plantar wart

261. In pregnancy deficiency anemia is all except:

a. Iron deficiency anemia

b. Folic acid deficiency anemia

c. Protein deficiency anemia

d. Bone marrow insufficiency

262. Features of true labor are following except:

a. Painful uterine contractions

b. Pain confined to lower abdomen

c. Formation of bag of water

d. Progressive effacement and dilatation of cervix

263. Norplant is a:

a. Progestin only delivery system containing levonorgestril

b. Oestrogen only delivery syatem containing levonorgestril

c. Combined delivery system containing levonorgestril

d. None

264. The causes arrest of after coming head of breech at the brim are all except:

a. Hydrocephalus

b. Deflexed head

c. Premature baby

d. Contracted pelvis

265. Foetal attitude is:

a. Relationship of the long axis of the foetus to the long axis of mother

b. Relation of foetal parts to each other

c. The part of the fetus that lies in the lower pole of uterus

d. The most dependent part of the fetus

266. At term of lower segment of uterus is made up of:

a. 30 % isthmus & 70% cervix

b. 50 % isthmus & 50% cervix

c. 70 % isthmus & 30% cervix

d. 75 % isthmus & 25% cervix

267. Blastocyst stage is:

a. 30-200 cells

b. 40-400 cells

c. 50-500 cells

d. 60 – 600 cells

268. Haemorrhage within 24 hrs of injury is known as:

a. Primary haemorrhage

b. Secondary haemorrhage

c. Reactionary haemorrhage

d. Chronic haemorrhage

269. Cause of gas gangrene:

a. Clostridium welchi

b. C. oedematous

c. C. septicum

d. All

270. Fourncer's gangrene ka taluq hai:

a. Gangrene of small intestine

b. Gangrene of big toe

c. Gangrene of genital area

d. Gangrene of caecum

271. Mc evedy operation fataq ki kis qism mei kiya jata hai?

a. Inguinal

b. Femoral

c. Umblical

d. Hiatus

272. Trans pyloric plane guzarta hai:
a. T12-L1 se
b. L5 – S1 se
c. T 10 se
d. L1 – L2 se

273. Tidy wounds are characterized by:
a. Contaminated tissue
b. Incised edges
c. Devitalised tissue present
d. Often tissue loss

274. Which is not a feature of C.B.D stone:
a. Pain
b. Fever
c. Jaundice
d. Septic shock

275. Charcot's triad is:
a. Jaundice with fever and vomiting
b. Jaundice with pain & fever
c. Pain with fever and vomiting
d. Pain with burning micturition and fever

276. What is Australia antigen?
a. HBc Ag
b. HBe Ag
c. HBs Ag
d. None

277. The characteristic feature of poisoning from "BEESH"
a. Tingling and numbness all over the body
b. Excessive salivation
c. Erythematous urtical rashes all over body
d. Raised blood pressure

278. Which of the following drug is not bactericidal drug?
a. Rifampacin
b. Isoniazid
c. Streptomycin
d. Ethambutol

279. Hepatitis B vaccine is:
a. Live attenuated vaccine
b. Inactivated vaccine
c. Toxoid
d. Cellular fraction

280. Vegetable hairs are:
a. Vegetable irritant
b. Mechanical irritant
c. Metallic irritant
d. Inorganic irritant

281. 16 yrs of age of a female is an age to give valid consent for:
a. Marriage contract
b. Lawful sexual intercourse
c. Majority

d. Employment

282. Hostile witness is one who:
a. Does not tell truth
b. Does not submit facts
c. Contradicts his own statement previously given
d. None

283. Narm hathon ya narm kapdon se malish karne ko kahte hai:
a. Dalk khasn
b. Dalk layn
c. Dalk mutadil
d. Dalk imlas

284. Ma'jaid al jawahar ki behatreen mishal konsi hai?
a. Chasma ka paani
b. Barish ka paani
c. Kunwon ka paani
d. Ma'dni paani

285. Husr kahte hai:
a. Qolinj ko
b. Qabz ko
c. Bavaseer ko
d. Hichki ko

286. Intestinal obstruction ki alamaat hoti hai:
a. Poore batan par resonant sound
b. Constipation
c. Colicky pain

d. All

287. Megaloblastic anemia is caused by deficiency of:

a. Iron
b. Vitamin B 12
c. Vitamin C
d. All

288. Kayser Fleischer ring is characteristic of:

a. Pterygium
b. Scleritis
c. Hemochromatosis
d. Wilson's disease

289. Chronic wasting diseases with signs of three D's :

a. Scurvy
b. Berberi
c. Pellagra
d. Rickets

290. Dalk istardad ka aham maqsad:

a. Rutubat aslia ko tahleel hone se bachana
b. Dorane riyazat paida hone wale fuzlat ko tahleel karna
c. Khoon aor rooh ko aza ki taraf jazb karna
d. All

291. Bahr qalbi me nabz:

a. Sari wa mutwatar
b. Quwi wa mutwatar

c. Azeem wa mutwatar

d. Bati wa zaieef

292. More sensitive index of cardiac function is:

a. Cardiac output

b. Stroke volume

c. Ejection fraction

d. None

293. Ghiza ke baad hamam karne se kiya hota hai?

a. Badan me hazaal hota hai

b. Badan farba ho jat hai

c. Ghiza aza me juzb ni hoti

d. None

294. Darj zel mei konsa sabab zilkul ama'ka nahi hai:

a. Basoor ama

b. Zoaf ama

c. Tez safra

d. Balgham shur

295. A reversible change in which one adult cell type is replaced by another adult:

a. Anaplasia

b. Metaplasia

c. Hyperplasia

d. Atrophy

296. Chaksu ko mudabbir karte hi:

a. Baadyaan ke paani me josh dekar

b. Ajwayin ke paani me bhigokar

c. Aab lemon mei kharl kar ke

d. Arq gau zaban me bhigokar

297. Mazo ko mudabbir karte hai:

a. Teen shabana roz sirka mei bhigokar

b. Til ke teil me is qadr bhigoyen ki who khl jaye

c. Sheer gaou me josh dekar

d. Amal atfa'ke zariye

298. Goliyon ko moti jaisa chamkane ka aml kahlata hai:

a. Sheeqal

b. Ghilaf halami

c. Ghilaf qarni

d. Tilayi

299. Amal tas'eed ko kahte hai:

a. Granulation

b. Sublimation

c. Evaporation

d. None

300. Aml Shahaq ke zariye safoof banaya jata hai:

a. Zafran aor kateera ka

b. Zafran aor samag arbi ka

c. Zafran aor mastagi ka

d. Samag arbi aor loban ka

301. Very fine powder banaya jata hai:

a. 85 no. sieve se

b. 120 no. sieve se

c. 44/85 no. sieve se

d. 60 no. sieve se

302. Kis tabeeb ne jild ko aza e mufrad me shamil kiya hai?

a. Jalinoos

b. Rabban Tabri

c. Abu Sahal Maseehi

d. Ibn Sina

303. Khof ki halat mei kiya hota hai?

a. Inbisaat rooh

b. Inqibaaz rooh

c. Both

d. None

304. Ehatbaas ghair zaroori ka sabab nahi hai:

a. Madda ka ziyada miqdar me hona

b. Madda ka ghaleez hona

c. Majari ka kushadah hona

d. Dafia fuzlaat ki hajit

305. Murakkabat me chandi aor sone ka aoraq ki shamuliyat ka maqsad unka androon badan:

a. Munjazb hona hai

b. Ek chemical reaction karna hai

c. Ek catalyst ka kaam karna hai

d. Murakkab ko khush zaiqa aor khusnuma banana hai

306. tijarti paimana par arq hsil karne ke liye munasib aala hai:

a. Nal bhabhka/deg bhbhka

b. Hamam mai'ya /hamam nariya

c. Garbh jantar

d. Tariq lolbi

307. Amal kashateer istimaal hota hai:

a. Ailaoos me

b. Ehatbaas bol me

c. Warm masana mei

d. Su'al quniya me

308. Riyazat ki ibtida me kis tarah ki nabz hoti hai:

a. Quwi, Azeem, saree aor mutwatar

b. Quwi, Sageer, saree aor mutwatar

c. Sageer, zaie'f , saree aor mutwatar

d. None

309. Ghiza lateef kaseerul taghzia ki misal hai:

a. Ma ul laham

b. Zardi baize neem barst

c. Angoor ka johar

d. All

310. Kaifiyat ke aeitbaar se dalk ki qism konsi hai?

a. Dalk kaseer

b. Dalk sulb

c. Dalk mutadil

d. All

311. Abraq kis azu ke liye muzir hai?

a. Gurda

B. Tihal

c. Both a & b

d. None

312. Zimad bawaseer ka juz khas hai:

a. Safeda qalai

b. Post beikh kbr

c. Zangar

d. Aqarqarha

313. Konsi dawa zamid nahi hai:

a. Nufooq

b. Ghalia

c. Wajoor

d. Furzaja

314. Bajra ki nabeez kahlati hai:

a. Nabeez al zarah

b. Nabeez al dakhn

c. Nabeez al wadi

d. None

315. Konsi dawa taqleel bol paida karti hai:

a. Qahwa

b. Tukhm khayareen

c. Sang sarmahi

d. Kundur

316. Hadtaal ka mutradif hai:

a. Shamul arz

b. Hujr abyaz

c. Hujr arzaq

d. Kasrul arz

317. Safed rang ka muslas chapta pathar kis se hasil hota hai:
a. Zagar se
b. Regmahi se
c. Safool naami machli se
d. Karm aroosak se

318. Habisud dam dawa ki shinakht kijeye:
a. Mochras
b. Narjeel dariyayi
c. Zoofa khusk
d. None

319. Medah lakdi ka nabati naam hai:
a. Abies pindrow
b. Hyssopus officinalis
c. Listea glutinosa
d. None of the above

320. Jamiul jawami'a kis tabeeb ki tasneef hai:
a. Hkm Baqa khan
b. Hkm Akbararzani
c. Hkm alvi khan
d. Hkm Ajmal khan

321. Mezan tib kiski tasneef hai:
a. Akbar arzani
b. Muhd Hussain Shirazi
c. Hkm Zaka khan
d. Hkm Wasil khan

322. Husr kahte hai:
a. Qolinj ko
b. Qabz ko
c. Bawaseer ko
d. Hichki ko

323. Intestinal obstruction ki alamaat hoti hai:
a. Resonant sound on whole abdomen
b. Constipation
c. Colicky pain
d. All of the above

324. Megaloblastic anemia is caused by deficiency of?
a. Iron
b. Vitamin B12
c. Vitamin C
d. All of the above

325. Kayser Fleischer ring is characteristic of:
a. Pterygium
b. Scleritis
c. Hemochromatosis
d. Wilson's disease

326. Chronic wasting disease with signs of 3 D's ?
a. Scurvy
b. Beriberi
c. Pellagra
d. Rickets

327. Dalk istardad ka aham maqsad hai:

a. Rutubat aslia ko tahleel hone se bachana

b. Dorane riyazat paida hone wale fuzlat ko tahleel karna

c. Khoon aor rooh ko aza ki taraf jazb karna

d. All of the above

328. Bahr qalbi mei nabz hoti hai:

a. Sari wa mutwatir

b. Qawi wa mutwatir

c. Azeem wa mutwatir

d. Bati wa zai'ef

329. More sensitive index of cardiac function is:

a. Cardiac output

b. Stroke volume

c. Ejection fraction

d. None of the above

(EXPLAINATION: More sensitive index of cardiac function is the EJECTION FRACTION, i.e., the ratio of stroke volume to end-diastolic volume (normal value = 67 ± 8%), which is frequently depressed in systolic heart failure, even when the stroke volume itself is normal.)

330. Ghiza ke baad hammam karne se kya hota hai?

a. Badan me hizaal hota hai

b. Badan farba hojata hai

c. Ghiza aza me jazb nahi hoti

d. None of the above

331. Darjzel me konsa sabab zalqul am'a ka nahi hai:

a. Basoor am'a

b. Zoa'f am'a

c. Tez safra

d. Balgham sour

332. Comedones kis marz me paye jate hai:

a. Scabies

b. Acne vulgaris

c. Vitiligo

d. Leprosy

333. Chronic Paronychia is mainly due to:

a. Candidal infection

b. Viral infection

c. Only bacterial infection

d. Protozoal infection

334. Lichenfied plaque due to repeated rubbing as a habit or in response to stress may be the feature of:

a. Lichen simpilex

b. Lichen planus

c. Atopic dermatitis

d. Eczema

(EXPLAINATION: This describes a plaque of lichenified eczema due to repeated rubbing or scratching as a habit or in response to stress.

Common sites include the neck, lower legs, and the ano-genital areas.)

335. Bars aor uski mujarrab dawa hai:

a. Jild par safed ma'il dhabbe – tukhm babchi wa atrilal

b. Jild par siyahi ma'il dhabbe – Ard baqla, ard Krishna

c. Jild par safed dhabbe- Tukhm babchi wa Atrilal

d. Jild par surkh dhabbe- Ard baqla, ard Krishna

336. Garam mammalik mei, garam aoqat par garam mizaj logon mei khastor par pasina ki kasrat hone par jild par hone wale chote chote kante daar daane alama'at ho sakti hai:

a. Hikka ki

b. Basoor saghar ki

c. Basoor labnia ki

d. Hisf ki

337. Which of the following is ectoparasitic infestation:

a. pediculosis & scabies

b. Pediculosis & mononucleosus

c. Pediculosis & leishmaniasis

d. All of the above

(EXPLAINATION: An ectoparasitic infestation is a parasitic disease caused by organisms that live primarily on the surface of the host. Examples: Scabies, Crab louse (pubic lice), Pediculosis (head lice), Lernaeocera branchialis.)

338. Marz qoba jism ke kin hisson ko mutasir karta hai:
a. Baalo'n aor nakhoon ko
b. Chehre aor sar ki jild ko
c. Kanjraan ko
d. All of the above

339. Complications of twin pregnancy during labour are following except:
a. Prolonged labour
b. Cord prolapsed
c. Post-partum haemorrhage
d. Sub involution

340. On the basis of the shape of inlet; female pelvis is divided into the following except:
a. Gynaecoid
b. Platypoid
c. Anthropoid
d. Android

341. Murabba sandal se muraad hai:
a. Sandal surkh ki lakdi ka murabba
b. Sandal safed ki lakdi ka murabba
c. Both
d. None

342. Qar'a ambaiq ka hindi naam hai:
a. Teju jantar
b. Luk jantar
c. Both

d. None

343. Maqtaar kiya hai:

a. Ek khas qism ki shishi jisme syal dawa rakhi jati hai

b. Ek khas qism ki qainchi jisse dawaon ko kata jata hai

c. Ek khas qism ka aala jisse qurs banaye jate hai

d. None

344. Dawsazi me DILUENTS ka istemaal hota hai:

a. Syrup ko banane me

b. Tablet banane mei

c. Ointment banane mei

d. Liniment banane mei

(**EXPLAINATION:** Diluents are also very important in the pharmaceutical industry. They are inactive ingredients that are added to tablets and capsules in addition to the active drug.)

345. Sahi jumla hai:

a. Creams neem jamid emulsion hai

b. Pastes marham ki ek khas qism hai

c. Pastes me ghair munhal ajza ki miqdar bahut ziyada hoti hai

d. All are correct

346. Sangrahni mei makhsoos tor par mufeed hai:

a. Asnasiya

b. Asirul maluk

c. Malti basnat

d. Anqarooya

347. Mufarrah sheikhur raies ka juz khas hai:
a. Darwanj aqrabi
b. Abresham
c. Marwareed
d. Musk wa ambar

348. Ball mill ka istemal hota hai:
a. Safoof sazi mei
b. Kushta sazi mei
c. Amal tajfeef mei
d. Amal taqteer me

349. Tar kharl karne ke aml ko kahte hai:
a. Levigation
b. Pulverization
c. Emulsification
d. Exsiccation

(EXPLAINATION: Levigation is the process of grinding an insoluble substance to a fine powder, while wet. The material is introduced into the mill together with water, in which the powdered substance remains suspended, and flows from the mill as a turbid liquid or thin paste, according to the amount of water employed. **Pulverization** is to reduce (a substance) to fine particles, as by crushing or grinding, or (of a substance) to be so reduced. **Emulsification** a process in which an emulsion is formed, an emulsion being a liquid containing fine droplets of another liquid without forming a solution, for example, fat droplets are emulsified in milk. **Exsiccation** is the process of being dried up; desiccation.)

350. Deedan am'a kis tarah ka marz hai:
a. Marz mujari
b. Marz miqdar
c. Marz adad
d. Marz waza'a

351. All are causes of avascular necrosis except:
a. Long term steroid therapy
b. Chronic alcoholism
c. Radiation therapy
d. Fungal infection

(EXPLAINATION: Mnemonics for the causes of avascular necrosis (AVN) or more correctly "osteonecrosis": STARS, PLASTIC RAGS, ASEPTIC.

STARS:
S: steroids
T: trauma (e.g. femoral neck fracture, hip dislocation, scaphoid fracture)
A: alcohol abuse
R: radiation osteonecrosis
S: sickle cell disease

PLASTIC RAGS
P: pancreatitis, pregnancy
L: lupus
A: alcohol

S: steroids
T: trauma
I: idiopathic, infection
C: caisson disease, collagen vascular disease
R: radiation, rheumatoid arthritis
A: amyloid arthropathy
G: Gaucher disease
S: sickle cell disease
ASEPTIC
A: alcohol
S: sickle cell disease / SLE
E: exogenous steroid
P: pancreatitis
T: trauma
I: infection
C: caisson disease)

352. A reversible change in which one adult cell type is replaced by another adult cell type is:
a. Anaplasia
b. Metaplasia
c. Hyperplasia
d. Atrophy

353. Causes of haemolytic anaemia are:
a. Extracorpuscular
b. Intrinsic
c. Environmental
d. Extracorpuscular & intracorpuscular both

d. Environmental

354. Chaksu ko mudabbir karte hai:

a. Baadyan ke paani mei josh dekar

b. Ajwayin ke paani mei bhigokar

c. Aab lemo me kharl karke

d. Arq gao zaban me bhigokar

355. Mazu ko mudabbir karte hai:

a. Teen shabana roz sirka mei bhigokar

b. Til ke tel mei isqadr bhigoye ki woh khil jaye

c. Sher gau me josh dekar

d. Aml atf'a ke zariye

356. Goliyon ko moti ke jaisa chamkane ka amal kahlata hai:

a. Saiql

b. Ghilaf halami

c. Ghilaf qarni

d. Tilayi

357. Amal tas'eed ko kahte hai:

a. Granulation

b. Sublimation

c. Evaporation

d. None

358. Amal shahaq ke zariye safoof banaya jata hai:

a. Zafran aor kateera ka

b. Zafran aor samag arbi ka

c. Zafran aor mastagi ka

d. Samag arbi aor loban ka

359. Ek very fine powder banaya jata hai:
a. Ek 85 no. sieve se
b. 120 no. sieve se
c. 44/85 no. sieve se
d. 60 no. sieve se

360. All the following structures are present in the carpal tunnel except:
a. Tendon of Palmaris longus
b. Tendon of flexor pollicis longus
c. Tendons of flexor digitorum profundus
d. Median nerve

361. All of the following muscles extend thigh at hip joint except:
a. Semitendinosus
b. Semimembranosus
c. Hamstring portion of aductor magnus
d. Gluteus medius

362. Ceruminous glands are found in which of the following structure:
a. Nose
b. Ear
c. Eye
d. Anus

363. Which of the following is the independent bone of the nose?
a. Inferior concha
b. Middle concha

c. Superior concha

d. Nasal septum

364. Fissure in ano is caused by one of the following condition:

a. Anal abscess

b. Rupture of anal valves

c. Internal piles

d. External piles

365. Pain sensation is carried by which of the following nerve fibres?

a. A

b. C

c. Both a & b

d. None

(EXPLAINATION: Group C nerve fibers are one of three classes of nerve fiber in the central nervous system and peripheral nervous system. The C group fibers are unmyelinated and have a small diameter and low conduction velocity. They include Postganglionic fibers in the autonomic nervous system (ANS), and nerve fibers at the dorsal roots (IV fiber). These fibers carry sensory information.

Damage or injury to nerve fibers causes neuropathic pain. Capsaicin activates C fibers Vanilloid receptors, giving chili peppers a hot sensation.**)**

366. Sympathetic preganglionic neurons secrete:

a. Acetylcholine

b. Nor epinephrine

c. GABA

d. None of the above

367. Peptic ulcer is caused due to infection of:

a. H. Influenza

b. Helico bacter pylori

c. Staphyloccus

d. Pneumocystis carini

368. Kernicterus is caused due to accumulation of bilirubin in:

a. Spleen

b. Liver

c. Brain

d. Kidney

369. Sabaat ka sabab hai:

a. Burudat ka ghalba

b. Rutubat ka ghalba

c. Badan me khoon ki kasrat

d. All of the above

370. Faras'al bol me mufeed hai:

a. Gulqand usli

b. Ma'ul asl

c. ma'ul shai'r

d. ma'ul jabn

371. Istifrag se qabl nuzij:

a. Zaroori hai

b. Ghair zarori hai

c. Sirf ghalba safra me ghair zarori hai

d. Nujiz ke bagair istifragh ba'z surto me wajib hai

372. Amraz bah me mareezon ke liye qabz ki behatreen dawa hai:

a. Sana makki

b. Turbud

c. Saqmoonia

d. Ispgol musallim

373. Dawa'al moz mustamil hai:

a. Zatur riya mei

b. Zatul janb mei

c. Shaheeqa mei

d. Shaqeeqa mei

374. Qalbi ghashi ka sabab hota hai:

a. Qalb ka warm haar

b. Qalb ka imtila

c. Qalb ka warm muzmin

d. Qalb ka sudda

375. Zagatudam ki surat me konsi tadbeer nafa hai:

a. Idrar

b. Fasd

c. Tariq

d. All

376. Warjish se qbl badan ko warjish ke liye amadah karne wli malish ko kahte hai:

a. Dalak istardad

b. Dalak istadad

c. Dalak khasn

d. Dalak imlas

377. Kis marz me fasd mamnuh hai:

a. Suda'a damwi

b. Qabz dai'mi

c. Arqunnisha

d. All

378. Fasd nahi kholna chahiye:

a. Jab jigar wa meda kamjor ho

b. Barid ratab amraz mei

c. both

d. None

379. All the muscles of tongue are supplied by the hypoglossal nerve except:

a. Genioglossus

b. Hyoglossus

c. Palatoglossus

d. Styloglossus

380. Regarding the spleen the following statement is true except that:

a. It is situated in right hypochondrium

b. It is a large lymphoid organ

c. It is supplied by the splenic artery

d. Its visceral surface is related to left kidney

381. The superior oblique muscle of eye ball is supplied by:
a. Trochlear nerve
b. Occulomotor nerve
c. Abducent nerve
d. Trigeminal nerve

382. Following arteries supply the medulla oblongata except:
a. Basilar artery
b. Posterior inferior cerebellar artery
c. Anterior inferior cerebellar artery
d. Anterior spinal artery

(EXPLAINATION: Blood to the medulla is supplied by a number of arteries.

Anterior spinal artery: This supplies the whole medial part of the medulla oblongata.

Posterior inferior cerebellar artery: This is a major branch of the vertebral artery, and supplies the posterolateral part of the medulla, where the main sensory tracts run and synapse. It also supplies part of the cerebellum.

Direct branches of the vertebral artery: The vertebral artery supplies an area between the other two main arteries, including the solitary nucleus and other sensory nuclei and fibers.)

383. Maqala abdaal advia al mustamila ki tasneef hai:

a. Zakriya Razi

b. Jalinoos

c. Ibn sina

d. Hkm ajmal khan

384. Aqaqiya ki muddat hayat hai:

a. 1 yr

b. 2 yrs

c. 5 yrs

d. 10 yrs

385. Habbul mumsik kiska mutradif naam hai:

a. Musk

b. Zafran

c. Musk dana

d. All

386. Badawardah kiya hai:

a. Mafroos booti

b. Darakht

c. Poda

d. Jhadi daar poda

387. Habbul qatn kiska mutradif naam hai:

a. Kalonji

b. Zeerah

c. Badam

d. Pamba daana

388. Bao badang ka mizaj kiya hai:

a. Haar yabis

b. Haar ratab

c. Barid yabis

d. Barid ratab

389. Isinglass kiya hai:

a. Reg maahi

b. Saresaham maahi

c. Kaf darya

d. None

390. Narkachoor kiya hai:

a. Zarnibaad

b. Zanjabel

c. Zarnab

d. Zarshak

391. Darjzel me konsi dawa "madah hayat" kahlati hai:

a. Khameera abresham hkm arsad wala

b. Dawa al misk mutadil

c. Majum falasfa

d. Tiryaq arba

392. Majum kakanj darjzel mei kis marz ki makhsoos dawa hai:

a. Dard hai' qolinj

b. Sara

c. Malikholya maraqi

d. Quruh gurda wa masana

393. Huziz maki kis pode se hasil kiya jata hai:

a. Shorea robusta

b. Berberis aristata

c. Smilax ornata

d. Doranicum hookerii

394. Dawali kahte hai:

a. Dorane sar ko

b. Pindli aor qadm ki rag ke phail jane ko

c. Khusiya ke rag ke phail jane ko

d. Jigar ki rag ke phail jane ko

395. Riya ke qarhe ko kahte hai:

a. Sil

b. Zatur riya

c. Diq

d. None

396. Ustusqa ka aam sabab hai:

a. Hazm medi ka zoaf

b. Hazm mevi ka zoaf

c. Hazm kabdi ka zoaf

d. All

397. Which of the following causes mouth ulcers:

a. Candidiasis

b. Measles

c. Behcet's disease

d. All

398. Development of Q waves in ECG suggestive of:

a. Angina pectoris

b. Ventricular fibrillation

c. Atrial fibrillation

d. Myocardial infarction

399. Kaifiyat ke aitbaar se dalak ki qism ki nishndehi kijeye:

a. Dalak kaseer

b. Dalak mutadil

c. Dalak sulb

d. All

400. Ishaal mei konsi tadbeer sabse behtar hai:

a. Hammam aor badan ki malish

b. Aaram ki nind

c. Shikam pe hijama lagana

d. None

Answer key AMU 2015 & 2016:

1. d, 2.d, 3. a, 4.a, 5.c, 6. b, 7. d, 8.a, 9.a, 10.a, 11. a, 12. a, 13.a, 14.a, 15.a, 16.a, 17.a, 18.c, 19.d, 20.a, 21. c, 22.a, 23.b, 24.c, 25.a, 26. b, 27.a, 28.d, 29.b, 30.d, 31.a, 32.d, 33.c', 34.b, 35.a, 36.a, 37.c, 38.b, 39.b, 40.b, 41.d, 42.b, 43.b, 44.b, 45.a, 46.a, 47.b, 48.d, 49.c, 50.b, 51.d, 52.c, 53.a, 54.a, 55.b, 56.c, 57.c, 58.b, 59.a, 60.a, 61. b, 62.d, 63.c, 64.a, 65.a, 66.a, 67..68.a, 69.a, 70.d, 71.c, 72.a, 73.b, 74.d, 75.c, 76.a, 77.c, 78.a, 79.a, 80.a, 81.d, 82.b, 83.b, 84.a, 85.c, 86.d, 87.d, 88.c, 89.a, 90.d, 91.d, 92.a, 93.b, 94.d, 95.d, 96.a, 97.a, 98.b, 99.c, 100.d, 101.b, 102.b, 103.a, 104.d,105.c, 106.b, 107.c, 108.b,109.b, 110.c, 111.a, 112.c, 113.a, 114.c, 115.a, 116.b, 117.b, 118.d, 119.d, 120.a, 121.b, 122.a, 123.a, 124.a, 125.c, 126.d, 127.c, 128.b, 129.a, 130.b, 131.a, 132.c, 133.c, 134.c, 135.a, 136.c, 137.d, 138.a, 139.d, 140.a, 141.d, 142.a, 143.a, 144.d, 145.c, 146.a, 147.a, 148.c, 149.d, 150.b, 151.a, 152.d, 153.b, 154.a, 155.d, 156.a, 157.d, 158.c, 159.a, 160.c, 161.d, 162.c, 163.a, 164.b, 165.b, 166.b, 167.d, 168.d, 169.c, 170.a, 171.c, 172.a, 173.b, 174.d, 175.c, 176.a, 177.d, 178.d, 179.c, 180.d, 181.c, 182.c, 183.a, 184.a, 185.c, 186.a, 187.c, 188.c, 189.a, 190.d, 191.c, 192.b, 193.c, 194.d, 195.c, 196.d, 197.a, 198.c, 199.d, 200.c, 201.c, 202.d, 203.a, 204.c, 205.d,

206.d, 207.b, 208.b, 209.c, 210.c, 211.c, 212.c, 213.c, 214.d, 215.b, 216.a, 217.c, 218.a, 219.a, 220.c, 221.d, 222.d, 223.d, 224.d, 225.d, 226.d, 227.c, 228.b, 229.d, 230.d, 231.c, 232.a, 233.b, 234.d, 235.b, 236.a, 237.c, 238. D, 239.b, 240.d, 241.b, 242.c, 243.a, 244.d, 245.a, 246.b, 247.c, 248.d, 249.d, 250.b, 251.d, 252.c, 253.b, 254.a, 255.b, 256.c, 257.d, 258.d, 259.d, 260.b, 261.d, 262.b, 263.c, 264.c, 265.b, 266.c, 267.a, 268.c, 269.a, 270.c, 271.b, 272.a, 273.b, 274.d, 275.c, 276.c, 277.a, 278.d, 279.a, 280.b, 281.b, 282.d, 283.d, 284.a, 285.b, 286.d, 287.a, 288.d, 289.c, 290.d, 291.c, 292.c, 293.b, 294.b, 295.b, 296.a, 297.b, 298.a, 299.b, 300.c, 301.b, 302.c, 303.b, 304.c, 305.d, 306.b, 307.b, 308.a, 309.d, 310.b, 311.c, , 312.a, 313.c, 314.c, 315.d, 316.c, 317.c, 318.d, 319.d, 320.c, 321.a, 322.b, 323.d, 324.a, 325.a, 326.c, 327.d, 328.c, 329.c, 330.b, 331.b, 332.b, 333.a, 334.b, 335.c, 336.d, 337.a, 338.d, 339.d, 340.b, 341.c, 342.a, 343.c, 344.b, 345.d, 346.c, 347.a, 348.a, 349.a, 350.c, 351.d, 352.b, 353.b, 354.a, 355.b, 356.a, 357.b, 358.c, 359.b, 360.a, 361.c, 362.b, 363.a, 364.a, 365.b, 366.a, 367.b, 368.c, 369.d, 370.d, 371.d, 372.d, 373.c, 374.b, 375.d, 376.b, 377.b, 378.c, 379.c, 380.b, 381.a, 382.c, 383.a, 384.c, 385.c, 386.c, 387.d, 388.a, 389.b, 390.a, 391.c, 392.d, 393.c, 394.b, 395.a, 396.c, 397.d, 398.d, 399.c, 400.c

ALL INDIA AYUSH POST GRADUATE ENTRANCE TEST 2019

1. In which disease Charcot leyden crystals are found in sputum in microscopic examination?

A. Pneumonia
B. Pulmonary tuberculosis
C. Bronchial asthma
D. Emphysema

Ans: C

Explanation:- Charcot–Leyden crystals are microscopic crystals made up of eosinophil protein galectin-10 and seen in people who have allergic reactions (asthma, bronchitis, allergic rhinitis and rhinosinusitis) and parasitic infections such as Entamoeba histolytica, Necator americanus, and Ancylostoma duodenale. Charcot–Leyden crystals are often seen pathologically in patients with bronchial asthma.

2. In which disease stool is associated with fat or oil like substances?

A. Hepatitis
B. Pancreatitis
C. Cholecystitis
D. Gastritis

Ans: B

3. Which of the following is NOT the finding of the urine of pregnant woman?

A. Aab-e Nakhood like colour
B. Cloud like froth
C. In the middle Qutn-e manfoosh like precipitate
D. "Ghee" like smell

Ans: D

4. Which of the following is an animal origin drug?

A. Hiran Khuri
B. Shaakhe Marjan
C. Ikleelul Malik
D Shehme Hanzal

Ans: B

5. What is the most common complication of undescended testis?

A. Sterility
B. Torsion of testis
C. Associated indirect inguinal hernia
D. Testicular Atrophy

Ans: C

Explanation:- Inguinal hernia. This is a weakened area in the lower belly wall or inguinal canal where intestines may push through. However, Infertility is most common when both testes don't descend.

6. The first dose of pentavalent vaccine is given at:

A. At birth
B. 6 Weeks
C. 9 Weeks
D. 14 Weeks

Ans: B

Explanation:- The pentavalent vaccine protects against five potential killers – Diptheria, Tetanus, Pertusis, Haemophilus influenzae type B vaccine (Hib), and Hepatitis B. This vaccine is available in various forms of liquid and lyophilised. However, under the UIP in India, the vaccine is available as a liquid formulation only. This vaccine comes in a liquid form in a vial which contains 10 doses. Each dose is 0.5 ml to be given by intra muscular injection in anterolateral aspect of the mid-thigh.

7. Which symptom remains dominant in *Warm-e - jigar Mohaddab*?

A. Hiccup
B. Vomiting
C. Loss of appetite

D. Shortness of breath
Ans: D

8. Scopolamine's action is:

A. Anti-pyretic
B. Anti-emetic
C. Analgesic
D. Anti-inflammatory

Ans: B

9. Norplant is related to:

A. Water purification
B. Contraception
C. Vaccine
D. Sanitation

Ans: B

10. Incidence rate is measured by:

A. Case control study
B. Cohort study
C. Cross sectional study
D. Cross over study

Ans: B

Explanation:- The measure of disease in cohort studies is the incidence rate, which is the proportion of subjects who develop the disease under study within a specified time period. The numerator of the rate is the number of diseased subjects and the denominator is usually the number of person-years of observation. The incidence rates for exposed and non-exposed subjects are calculated separately.

11. Clinical feature of "*Fasad-e- Shahwat*' is:

A. Decreased appetite
B. Loss of appetite
C. Desire to eat sweet things
D. Desire to eat bad things

Ans: D

12. Migratory polyarthritis is the feature of:

A. Rheumatic arthritis
B. Rheumatoid arthritis
C. Osteoarthritis
D. Gouty arthritis

Ans: A

Explanation:- Migratory arthritis occurs when pain spreads from one joint to another. In this type of arthritis, the first joint may start to feel better before pain starts in a different joint.

13. Dry Semen stains on clothes are identified by:

A. Spectroscopy
B. Ultraviolet light
C. Infrared rays
D. Magnifying lens

Ans: B

Explanation:- UV light/rays for seminal stains and infrared rays for old blood stains.

14. Absolute inability to perform sexual act is called:

A. Aqoona
B. Ananiyat
C. Farismoos
D. Azyoot
Ans: B

15. Which of the following drug is *Mushil sauda*?

A. Turbud
B. Suranjan
C. Saqmoonia
D. Ghariqoon

Ans: D

16. Postpartum haemorrhage may cause:

A. HELLP Syndrome

B. Asherman syndrome
C. Sheehan syndrome
D. Couvelair uterus

Ans: C

Explanation:- Sheehan syndrome is also called postpartum hypopituitarism. It is is a condition that happens when the pituitary gland is damaged during childbirth. It's caused by excess blood loss (hemorrhage) or extremely low blood pressure during or after labor.

17. Which of the following is not an ingredient of arq e ajeeb?

A. Jauhar e Gilo
B. Jauhar e podina
C. Jauhar e Ajwain
D. Kafoor

Ans: A

18. Which of the following does NOT cause airway narrowing in an asthma attack?

A. Destruction of airway
B. Mucus hyper secretion
C. Airway oedema
D. Bronchospasm

Ans: A

19. Tri matter theory was presented by:

A. Aesculapius
B. Hippocrates
C. Razi
D. Ibn Sina

Ans: B

20. Name the organ where the sinusoids are present:

A. Brain
B. Liver
C. Heart
D. Skin

Ans: B

21. For the disease Niqris, which is <u>incorrect</u>:

A. Affects mostly the rich people
B. Affects the joints of finger
C. Affects the bigger joints of body
D. Causative matter belongs to uric acid

Ans: C

22. Woods Lamp is used in the examination of:

A. Eczema
B. Psoriasis
C. Leucoderma
D. Tinea
Ans: C

Explanation:- A Wood's lamp examination is a procedure that uses transillumination (light) to detect skin pigment disorders such as vitiligo. This test is also known as the black light test or the ultraviolet light test.

23. The commonest type of hypospadias is:

A. Coronal
B. Penile
C. Glandular
D. Penoscrotal
Ans: C

24. Diameter of placenta at full term is:

A. 10-15 cm
B. 15-20 cm
C. 20-25 cm
D. 25-30 cm

Ans: B

25. Commonest site of squamous cell carcinoma of vagina is:

A. Upper third anterior wall
B. Upper third posterior wall
C. Middle third
D. Lower third

Ans: B

26. Liquefaction necrosis is seen in:

A. Brain
B. Heart
C. Liver
D. Kidney

Ans: A

Explanation:- Liquefactive necrosis is a type of necrosis in which the dead tissue turns into a liquid substance. This condition usually occurs in the central nervous system, especially in the brain. When the cells die, they are digested by lysosomes in the body. This digestion process results in the formation of pus-filled cysts.

27. Chaksu is boiled in...in order to detoxify it:

A. Sirka
B. Arq Badiyan

C. Arq Mako
D. Arq Lemoo

Ans: B

28. Which is the first bone to ossify during foetal life?

A. Clavicle
B. Sternum
C. Humerus
D. Ulna

Ans: A

29. In which disease Negri bodies are seen?

A. Meningococcal meningitis
B. Neurocystocercosis
C. HIV
D. Rabies

Ans: D

Explanation:- The pathologic finding of RABIES in the central nervous system is the formation of cytoplasmic inclusions called negri bodies within neurons. Negri bodies are distributed throughout the brain, particularly in Ammon's horn, the cerebral cortex, the brain stem, the hypothalamus, the purkinje cells of the cerebellum and the dorsal spinal ganglia. (Park ed. 22, p.251)

30. Jauhar-e-Raskapoor is obtained by:

A. Amal-e-Tareeq
B. Amal-e-Taseed
C. Amal-e-Taqleem
D. Amal-e-Taghseel

Ans: B

31. What is the most common problem after prostatectomy?

A. Erectile dysfunction
B. Retrograde ejaculation
C. Prostatic haematuria
D. Severe sepsis

Ans: B

Explanation:- **Retrograde** ejaculation (ejaculation into the bladder rather than out of the penis).

32. Which of the following Massage prepares the body for exercise?

A. Dalak Isterdaad
B. Dalak Istedad
C. Dalak Khashan

D. Dalak Amlas

Ans: B

33. Most common complication of intercondylar fracture of Humerus is:

A. Malunion
B. Non-union
C. Stiffness of elbow
D. Osteoarthritis

Ans: C

34. According to whom, for Renal stones "Fa'ali sabab is heat and Maddi sabab is thick viscid fluid"?

A. Najeebuddin Samarqandi
B. Shaikh Bu Ali Sina
C. Jalinoos
D. Buqrat

Ans: A

35. "Intisab-un-nafas" is used for which disease?

A. Asthma
B. Pneumonia
C. Pleurisy
D. Pulmonary Tuberculosis

Ans: A

36. Active ingredient of Tiryaq-e- Nazla is:

A. Tukhm-e-Khashkhash
B. Post-e-Khashkhash
C. Bazrulbanj
D. Tukhm-e-Kahoo

Ans: B

37. What is the common congenital renal anomaly?

A. Horse shoe kidney
B. Polycystic kidney
C. Renal Ectopia
D. Duplication of pelvis

Ans: D

38. Scrotal tongue is a feature of:

A. Congenital hypothyroidism
B. Turner syndrome
C. Down syndrome
D. Measles

Ans: C

39. Ratio of Drug and Water in Arq should be:

A: 1:4
B. 1:8

C: 1:12
D. 1:16
Ans: D

40. Hepatitis C virus was identified in:

A. 1989
B. 1998
C. 1985
D. 1986

Ans: A

41. A child stands with support, speaks mama and has immature pincer grasp, what is the approximate age?

A. 6 months
B. 9 months
C. 01 year
D. 18 months

Ans: B

42. Activation of Vitamin D occurs in which of the following organ?

A. Heart
B. Kidney
C. Lung
D. Skin

Ans: B

43. *Amal-e-Tarseeb* is:

A. Fermentation
B. Sublimation
C. Sedimentation
D. Crystallization

Ans: C

44. Haemoptysis may be found in:

A. Tricuspid stenosis
B. Mitral stenosis
C. Endocarditis
D. Myocarditis

Ans: B

45. What is surface marking of superficial inguinal ring?

A. Just above pubic tubercle
B. Midway above inguinal ligament
C. Femoral triangle
D. At level of iliac triangle

Ans: A

46. Deficiency of which Vitamin is not known in new born?

A. Vitamin A
B. Vitamin D
C. Vitamin E
D. Vitamin K

Ans: C

47. Jules Guerin, a French physician in 1848 introduced:

A. Public health
B. Community medicine
C. Social Medicine
D. Preventive Medicine

Ans: C

48. Jadwar and Ude Saleeb are commonly used for which ailment?

A. Leucorrhoea
B. Hysteria
C. Uterine prolapsed
D. Pruritus vulva

Ans: B

49. Black tongue is seen in abuse of which drug?

A. Heroine
B. Dhatura

C. Smoking

D. Cocaine

Ans: D

50. Ulcerative colitis is classified as which one of the following types of disease?

A. Su-e-Tarkib

B. Su-e-Mizaj

C. Tafarruq-e-Itesal

D. Amraz-e-Miqdar

Ans: C

51. The first permanent tooth to erupt is:

A. Incisor

B. Canine

C. Premolar

D. Molar

Ans: A

52. Grey Turner's sign is seen in:

A. Acute Haemorrhagic pancreatitis

B. Acute Cholecystitis

C. Intestinal perforation

D. Pancreatic cyst

Ans: A

53. Which bone does not contain the red marrow?

A. Vertebrae
B. Ribs
C. Sternum
D. Clavicle
Ans: D

54. A person is said to be infertile when sperm count is less than?

A. 20 millions/ml
B. 40 millions/ml
C. 60 millions/ml
D. 80 millions/ml

Ans: A

55. Which type of Massage done for hardening the organs?

A. *Dalak-e-Layyen*
B. *Dalak-e-Sulb*
C. *Dalak-e-Kaseer*
D. *Dalak-e-Mutadil*
Ans: B

56. Which of the following is beneficial medicine for *Istisqa*?

A. Dawaul Kurkum

B. Dawaul Misk Motadil
C. Sharbat Faryadaras
D. Sharbat Neelofar

Ans: A

57. According to Buqrat, how many times should Qai can be induced in a month for Hifze Sehat?

A. Once
B. Twice
C. Thrice
D. Four times

Ans: B

58. Severe headache circumscribing whole head is called:

A. Suda Shaqeeqa
B. Suda Baiza wa Khooza
C. Suda Usaba
D. Suda Safravi

Ans: B

59. What is shape of epiglottic cartilage?

A. Leaf like
B. Ring like
C. Triangular
D. Square shaped

Ans: A

60. *Samm-e-Mutlaq* acts through its:

A. Kaifiyat
B. Kammiyat
C. Surat-e-Nauiya
D. Kammiyat wa kaifiyat

Ans: C

61. What is the cause of Hirschsprung's disease?

A. Hypokalaemia
B. Absence of ganglion cell in anorectum
C. Anal stenosis
D. Iliocaecal hyperplastic tuberculosis

Ans: B

Explanation: Hirschsprung's disease is a condition that affects the large intestine (colon) and causes problems with passing stool. It occurs when nerve cells in the colon don't form completely. Nerves in the colon control the muscle contractions that move food through the bowels. Without the contractions, stool stays in the large intestine.

62. After taking *Mushil* drugs, water should not be taken at least for:

A. 1 Hour

B. 2 Hours
C. 3 Hours
D. 4 Hours

Ans: D

63. In which disease patient walks in a haphazard way?

A. Subara
B. Mania
C. Kaboos
D. Qutrub

Ans: D

64. "One or few rashes with burning sensation and mild inflammation" is the symptoms of which disease?

A. Erysipelas
B. Herpes
C. Eczema
D. Carbuncle

Ans: B

65. "*Alkhajeel*" is used as synonym of which disease?

A. Gonorrhoea
B. Impotence

C. Syphilis

D. Premature ejaculation

Ans: C

66. Treatment of which disease is NOT similar to "*Baul Fil Farash*"?

A. Salasul Baul

B. Taqteerul Baul

C. Usrul Baul

D. Istirkhae-Masana

Ans: C

67. The sequence of treatment in *Zof-e-Bah* is:

A. Tahreek-Taqviyat-Taskeen

B. Taqviyat-Taskeen-Tahreek

C. Taskeen-Taqviyat-Tahreek

D. Taskeen-Tahreek-Taqviyat

Ans: C

68. Tall P-wave in ECG denotes:

A. Normal

B. Sign of ischaemia

C. Right atrial enlargement

D. Left atrial enlargement

Ans: C

69. Which of the following is vernacular name of Jadwar khatai?

A. Mahe-Rubiyaan
B. Mahe-Parveen
C. Mahe-Moorad
D. Mahe-Rajab

Ans: B

70. *Tafarruq e- ittesal* **of skin is called as:**

A. Sahaj
B. Kasar
C. Batar
D. Hatak

Ans: A

71. In case of menorrhagia, cupping is done at:

A. Lowe back
B. Below the breast
C. Below the umbilicus
D. Nape of the neck

Ans: B

72. In which of the following disorders jugular vein distention is most prominent?

A. Abdominal aortic aneurysm
B. Heart failure
C. Myocardial infarction
D. Pneumothorax

Ans: B

73. Usool-e-ilaj and drugs for *HIKKATUL MASHAIKH* may be:

A. Murattibat-Roghan badam Shirin
B. Mubarridat-Roghan kadu
C. Musakhkhinat- Roghan Bed Anjeer
D. Musaffiya-Chiraita

Ans: A

74. What is the actual cause of disease *Kaboos*?

A. Fasad-e-Khayal
B. Fasad-e-Hazm
C. Asaab ka Taa'sur
D. Sarsam

Ans: C

75. Tahabbuj is an example of:

A. Warm Saudawi
B. Warm Maai
C. Warm Reehi

D. Warm Sulb

Ans: C

76. Cheiloscopy is the study of prints of:

A. Mouth
B. Eyes
C. Nose
D. Lips

Ans: D

77. The chief ingredient of Majoon Fanjanosh is:

A. Ajwain Khorasani
B. Dhatura
C. Khabsul Hadeed
D. Asrol

Ans: C

78. Which of the following is inclined towards heat and dryness?

A. Balgham-e-Hamiz
B. Balgham-e-Malih
C. Balgham-e-Tafih
D. Balgham-e- Afis

Ans: B

79. Dalak Bawaqt-e-khawab comes under which type of Dalak?

A. Dalak Layyan
B. Dalak Isterdaad
C. Dalak Amlas
D. Dalak Khashin
Ans: B

80. The "term Basurrabasta" is particularly used with:

A. Kasni
B. Kasoos
C. Kasondi
D. Kaknaj
Ans: B

81. What is botanical name of *Jafte Baloot*?

A. Ipomea turpethum
B. Quericus incana
C. Quericus infectoria
D. Symplocos racemosa

Ans: B

82. Which of the following organ has the most moderate temperament?

A. Qalb

B. Azm
C. Jild
D. Shahm
Ans: C

83. Ligature mark of Hanging is a type of:

A. Linear abrasion
B. Graze abrasion
C. Pressure abrasion
D. Impact abrasion

Ans: C

84. Commonly found in females with phlegmatic temperament:

A. Dysmenorrhaea
B. Menorrhagia
C. Amenorrhoea
D. Leucorrhoea

Ans: C

85. How many conditions are required for experiment, as per Ibn Nafis?

A. 5
B. 7
C. 8
D. 9

Ans: B

86. Main action of Juntiyana drug is:

A. Musakkin
B. Haemostatic
C. Tiryaq Sumoom
D. Mufarreh

Ans: C

87. Chronic carrier state is seen in all EXCEPT:

A. Hepatitis-B
B. Diphtheria
C. Typhoid
D. Chicken pox

Ans: D

88. The length of the Bartholin's duct is approximately:

A. 10 mm
B. 20 mm
C. 30 mm
D. 40 mm

Ans: B

89. Which of the following is the composition of *Shatarul Ghib*?

A. Humma Ghib with Lisqa
B. Humma Ghib Lazima with Lisqa
C. Humma Ghib with Muwaziba
D. Humma Ghib Lazima with Muwaziba

Ans: A

90. Thyroid hormones belong to which class of hormones?

A. Steroids
B. Proteins
C. Polypeptides
D. Tyrosine derivative

Ans: D

91. Exuberant granulation tissue is seen in:

A. Sinus
B. Haemorrhoids
C. Rectal prolapsed
D. Fissure

Ans: A

92. *Aqaleem* (Regions) are how many?

A. Five
B. Six
C. Seven
D. Eight

Ans: C

93. Lumbar sympathectomy in Buerger's disease is usually done for:

A. Rest pain
B. Intermittent claudication
C. Skin ulcer
D. Foot gangrene

Ans: C

94. Which of the following alkaloids are found in *Azaraqi?*

A. Nyoscamine + Atropine
B. Scopolamine + Atropine
C. Strychnine + Brucine
D. Strychnine + Nicotine

Ans: C

95. In which of the fever Spleen is affected?

A. Humma Ghib
B. Humma Lisqa
C. Humma Muwaziba
D. Humma Ruba'a

Ans: D

96. Who was the first physician to discover pulmonary blood circulation?

A. Abul Qasim Zahravi
B. Najibuddin Samarqandi
C. Ibn Khtib
D. Ibn Nafis

Ans: D

97. Which of the following test is used for bile salt in urine?

A. Rothera's Test
B. Hay Test
C. Fauchet's Test
D. Ehrilich Test

Ans: B

98. Splenomegaly is an example of:

A. Amraz Shakal
B. Amraz Majari
C. Amraz Miqdar
D. Amraz Aoiya

Ans: C

99. Red-Glow translucency is seen in:

A. Hernia

B. Hydrocele
C. Omphalocele
D. Haematocele
Ans: B

100. Which muscle is called as Peripheral heart?

A. Soleus
B. Gartocnemius
C. Popliteus
D. Tibialis posterior
Ans: A

TEST YOUR KNOWLEDGE (MODERN ASPECT)

1. Deficiency of ------------ causes Goiter.
A: Potassium
B: Protein
C: Iodine
D: Vitamin K

2. What we use for snake bite.
A: Antibiotic
B: Anti fungal
C: Anti venom
D: Anti virus

3. What is gynaecomastia?
A. Flat chest in females.
B. Enlarged male breasts.
C. Female sterility.
D. Menstrual disorder.

4. During the replication of DNA, the synthesis of DNA on lagging strand takes place in segments, these segments are called:
A. Satellite segments
B. Double helix segments
C. Kornbeg segments
D. Okazaki segments

5. When preparing to reconstitute a drug from a powder form, the nurse should first.
A. Use sterile water

B. vigorously shake

C. follow directions on label for diluent to use

D. Discard the vital and the unused medication

6. The following are chromosomal abnormalities EXCEPT:

A. Down's syndrome.

B. Mendel's syndrome.

C. Turna's syndrome.

D. Klenefelter's syndrome.

7. Diabetes insipedus is caused by lack of??

A. ACTH

B. ADH

C. oxytocin

D. insulin

8. Over production of cortisol leads to...?

A. Addison's disease

B. Acromegaly

C. Epilepsy

D. Cushing's syndrome.

9. A genetically transmitted haemoglobin abnormality is:

A. Leukaemia

B. Hemophilia

C. Hematuria

D. Thalassaemia

**10. A client with B negative blood requires a blood transfusion during surgery. If no B negative blood

is available, the client should be transfused with:
A. A positive blood
B. B positive blood
C. O negative blood
D. AB negative blood

11. Dengue virus distroy ----- ?
A. RBCs
B. WBCs
C. Platelets
D. None

12. Emphysema is a disease that effect which part of the body.
A. lung
B. liver
C. heart
D. kidney

13. Vitamin K is prescribed for a neonate. A nurse prepares to administer the medication in which muscle site?
A. Deltoid
B. Triceps
C. Vastus lateralis
D. Biceps

14. Double vision is also known as:
A. myopia
B. hyperopia
C. presbyopia

D. Diplopia

15. Which of the following joint allow movement in only one direction?
A. pivot joint
B. gliding joint
C. hinge joint
D. Ball and socket joint

16. Which of the following statement is true regarding the visual changes associated with cataracts?
A. Both eyes typically cataracts at the same time
B. The loss of vision is experienced as a painless, gradual blurring
C. The patient is suddenly blind
D. The patient is typically experiences a painful, sudden blurring of vision.

17. Which of the following vitamin helps in normal formation of red blood cell and for health of nerve tissues?
A. Vitamin K
B. Vitamin C
C. Vitamin B12
D. Vitamin A

18. Which of the following symptoms is common in clients with TB?
A. Weight loss
B. Increased appetite

C. Dyspnea on exertion

D. Mental status changes

19. A client is suspected of developing diabetes insipidus. Which of the following is the most effective assessment?

A. Taking vital signs every 4 hours

B. Monitoring blood glucose

C. Assessing ABG values every other day

D. Measuring urine output hourly.

20. Travellers diarrhea is caused by mainly?

A. Clostridium perfringens.

B. Vibrio cholerae.

C. Shigellae.

D. Escherichia coli.

21. A nurse is caring for a male client with emphysema who is receiving oxygen. The nurse assesses the oxygen flow rate to ensure that it does not exceed:

A. 1 L/min

B. 2 L/min

C. 6 L/min

D. 10 L/min

22. A patient is admitted to the medical unit with possible Graves' disease (hyperthyroidism). Which assessment finding supports this diagnosis?

A. Periorbital edema

B. Bradycardia

C. Exophthalmos

D. Hoarse voice

23. Rothera's Test is for?

A. sugar

B. bile salt

C. acetone

D. albumin

24. A two month old infant is brought to the clinic for the first immunization against DPT. The nurse should administer the vaccine via what route?

A. Oral.

B. Intramascular

C. Subcutaneous

D. Intradermal

25. Pulmonary embolism is most closely related to?

A. Deep vein thrombosis

B. Collapsed lung

C. Hemophilia

D. Bronchitis

26. Which of following Vitamin is given at birth to prevent newborn baby from Bleeding?

A. Vitamin A

B. Vitamin B

C. Vitamin K

D. Vitamin D

27. Gallbladder inflammation is known as:
A. Cholecystitis
B. Asymphtomatia Bacteria
C. Urethritis
D. Pyelongephritis

28. Onset of menstrual cycle at the time of puberty is known as?
A. Menopause
B. Menarche
C. Menstruation
D. Metamerism

29. Circulation of blood that takes place between heart and lung is called?
A. systematic circulation
B. body circulation
C. Pulmonary circulation
D. Heart to lung circulation.

30. Projectile vomiting is the main feature of?
A. Gastritis
B. Duodenal ulcer
C. pyloric stenosis
D. Intusucception

31. Which of the following is NOT a risk factor for cardiovascular disease?
A. obesity
B. cigarette smoking

C. elevated blood cholesterol

D. consumption of aspirin.

32. The most common organ affected in subinvolution is .....

A. uterus

B. vagina

C. Breast

D. ovary.

33. 'Pap's smear test ' is used for screening of which of the following?

A. Breast cancer

B. Cervical cancer.

C. Ovarian cancer

D. Liver Cancer

34. Osteomalacia in adults is caused due to the deficiency of:

A. Vitamin A

B. Vitamin E

C. Vitamin D

D. Vitamin C

(**EXPLAINATION:** Osteomalacia is a weakening of the bones. Problems with bone formation or with the bone building process cause osteomalacia.

Osteomalacia isn't the same as osteoporosis. Osteoporosis is a weakening of living bone that has already been formed and is being remodeled.

Osteomalacia is most commonly caused by a lack of vitamin D. Vitamin D is an important nutrient that helps you absorb calcium in your stomach.

Vitamin D also helps maintain calcium and phosphate levels for proper bone formation. It's made within the skin from exposure to ultraviolet (UV) rays in sunlight. It can also be absorbed from foods like dairy products and fish.

Low levels of vitamin D mean that your body cannot process the calcium your bones need for structural strength. This can result from a problem with diet, lack of sun exposure, or a problem with your intestines.)

35. Neonates of mothers with diabetes are at risk for which complication following birth?
A. Atelectasis
B. Microcephaly
C. Pneumothorax
D. Macrosomia

(**EXPLAINATION:** Neonates of mothers with diabetes are at increased risk for macrosomia (excessive fetal growth) as a result of the combination of the increased supply of maternal glucose and an increase in fetal insulin.)

36. What term best describes a newly fertilized egg?
A. Zygote

B. Fetus

C. Embryo

D. Baby

(**EXPLAINATION:** A zygote is a eukaryotic cell formed by a fertilization event between two gametes. The zygote's genome is a combination of the DNA in each gamete, and contains all of the genetic information necessary to form a new individual. In multicellular organisms, the zygote is the earliest developmental stage.)

37. Enlargement of salivary gland is termed as?

A. siladenitis

B. sialadenoma

C. sialadenopathy

D. sialden

(**EXPLAINATION**: Painless enlargement of the salivary glands, occurring without findings that suggest salivary gland cancer, infection (sialadenitis), inflammation, or stone disease. It is most obvious in the parotid glands. Commonly associated conditions include alcoholic cirrhosis, breast feeding, diabetes mellitus, eating disorders, pregnancy, and malnutrition.)

38. What is angina?

A. A congenital heart disease

B. Inflammation of the heart muscle

C. Decrease in size of the heart

D. Chest pain from lack of oxygen

(EXPLAINATION: Angina is chest pain or discomfort caused when your heart muscle doesn't get enough oxygen-rich blood. It may feel like pressure or squeezing in your chest. and this may spread to your arms, neck, jaw, back or stomach as well.)

39. A patient is scheduled for a magnetic resonance imaging (MRI) scan for suspected lung cancer. Which of the following is a contraindication to the study for this patient?

A. The patient is allergic to shellfish.

B. The patient has a pacemaker.

C. The patient suffers from claustrophobia.

D. The patient takes anti-psychotic medication.

(EXPLAINATION: The implanted pacemaker will interfere with the magnetic fields of the MRI scanner and may be deactivated by them. Shellfish/iodine allergy is not a contraindication because the contrast used in MRI scanning is not iodine-based. Open MRI scanners and anti-anxiety medications are available for patients with claustrophobia. Psychiatric medication is not a contraindication to MRI scanning.)

40. A leukemia patient has a relative who wants to donate blood for transfusion. Which of the following donor medical conditions would prevent this?

A. A history of hepatitis C five years previously.
B. Cholecystitis requiring cholecystectomy one year previously.
C. Asymptomatic diverticulosis.
D. Crohn's disease in remission.

(EXPLAINATION: Hepatitis C is a viral infection transmitted through bodily fluids, such as blood, causing inflammation of the liver. Patients with hepatitis C may not donate blood for transfusion due to the high risk of infection in the recipient. Cholecystitis (gall bladder disease), diverticulosis, and history of Crohn's disease do not preclude blood donation.)

41. Thick yellow drainage from the wound is know as ....
A. sanguineus
B. serous sanguineus
C. serous
D. purulent

42. Which of the following is NOT a function of the kidneys?
A. Fluid and electrolyte balance
B. Maintenance of pH balance
C. Regulation of blood pressure
D. Production of adrenaline

43. Trachoma is the infection of?
A. skin

B. liver

C. eye

D. trachea

44. Instructions to take a medication "pc" means:

A. at bedtime

B. before meals

C. after meals

D. every morning

45. Egrocalciferol is also known as:

A. Vitamin A

B. Vitamin K

C. Vitamin E

D. Vitamin D

46. One of the following is known as physical antidote?

A. activated charcoal

B. potassium permagnet

C. tannic acid

D. milk of magnesia

47. Antitussive is indicated to:

A. encourage removal of secretions through coughing.

B. relieve rhinitis.

C. control a productive cough.

D. relieve a dry cough.

48. Torniquete test is indicated in diagnosis of:

A. hypertension

B. Deep venous thrombosis

C. filaria
D. Dengue.

49. Wilm's tumor is a condition affecting:
A. Kidney
B. Bone
C. Blood
D. Brain stem

(EXPLAINATION: Wilms tumor (also called nephroblastoma) is a type of cancer that starts in the kidneys. It is the most common type of kidney cancer in children.**)**

50. Bartholin duct present in the?
A. vagina
B. Penis
c. Mouth
D. Breast

(EXPLAINATION: The Bartholin's glands (also called greater vestibular glands) are two pea sized compound racemose glands located slightly posterior and to the left and right of the opening of the vagina. They secrete mucus to lubricate the vagina and are homologous to bulbourethral glands in males**.)**

51. Gestational diabetes occurs:
A During pregnancy
B After a bout with shingles
C At birth
D After menopause

52. Removal of gall bladder would lead to:
A. Impairment of digestion of fats
B. Impairment of digestion of protein
C. Jaundice
D. Increased acidity in intestine

53. Myasthenia gravis is a disease of:
A. Neuromuscular junction.
B. Anterior horn cells
C. Skeletal muscle
D. Spinal cord

54. What is commonly known as 'biological clock'?
A. Parathyroid gland
B. Adrenal gland
C. Pineal gland.
D. Thyroid gland

55. Which structure is also known as bregma?
A. Anterior fontanelle
B. Posterior fontanelle
C. Lambdoid suture
D. Frontal suture

56. Excessive iron storage in the body is called....?
A. hematochesia
B. hematochromatosis
C. pheresis
D. hemosiderosis

57. Phototherapy is used to treat newborns with:
A. Azotemia

B. Hyperbilirubinemia

C. Hypoglycemia

D. Premature delivery

58. After delivery, best time to start breast feeding is?

A. Within one hour

B. 6 hours

C. 24 hours

D. 36 hours

59. The route of administration for BCG vaccine?

A. i.v

B. i.m

(c) Intradermal

(d) Transdermal patch

60. What is neonatal period?

A. 1 to 3 years

B. 0 to 14 days

C. 1 weeks to 1month

D. 0 to 28days

61. Low secretion of glucocorticoid causes?

A. Addison's disease

B. Micromegaly

C. Cretinism

D. Dwarfism

62. Which anti tuberculin drug producess Red colour urine.......................... (its not haematuria it's only colour of that drug)

A. isonizide
B. rifampicin
C. ethambutol
D. pyridoxin.

63. Which of the following STD causes foetal abnormality?
A. Herpes
B. Hepatitis
C. Gonococci
D. Syphilis

64. Hypertensive disorders of pregnancy is:
A. Eclampsia
B. tachycardia
C. bradycardia
D. none of above

65. High fever, headache, skin rash & bright red spots are the symptoms of:
A. Small pox
B. Rabies
C. Mumps
D. Measles

66. Which vitamin deficiency is most commonly seen in a pregnant women who is on phenytoin therapy for epilepsy?
A. Vitamin-B6
B. Vitamin-B12

C. Vitamin-A

D. Folic acid

67. Test for hypersensitivity is called?

A. Patrick's test

B. Post-coital test

C. VDRL test

D. Patch test

68. Stiffness occur to the body after death is known as?

A. Livor Mortis

B. Rigor Mortis

C. Algor Mortis

D. Tardieu Spots

(EXPLAINATION: Rigor Mortis is the stiffening of the body after death because of a loss of Adenosine Triphosphate (ATP) from the body's muscles. ATP is the substance that allows energy to flow to the muscles and help them work and without this the muscles become stiff and inflexible**.)**

69. Which valve prevents the backwards flow of blood in to the left atrium?

A. Aortic valve

B. Pulmonary valve

C. Mitral valve

D. Tricuspid valve

70. Sengstaken-blakemore tube is use for?
A. portal hypertension
B. esophageal varices
C. peritoneovenous shunt
D. pericardiocentesis

(EXPLAINATION: The Sengstaken-Blakemore tube is used to treat upper gastrointestinal bleeding from esophageal varices. It is made of rubber and has two lumens used to inflate the gastric and esophageal balloons, with one tube reserved for gastric suction or drainage.**)**

71. During pregnancy the purplish discoloration of vaginal mucosa is known as?
A. Hegar's sign
B. Chadwick's sign
C. Ladin's sign
D. Goodell's sign

72. Mammary gland is type of?
A. Endocrine gland
B. Merocrine gland
C. Halocrine gland
D. Apocrine gland

73. Movement of fetus, felt by a pregnant women at 18-20 week of pregnancy is known as:-
A. lightening
B. Quickening

C. Amenorrhoea

D. Weaning

(**EXPLAINATION:** Quickening is the moment in pregnancy when the pregnant woman starts to feel or perceive fetal movements in the uterus.)

74. Asthmatic patients are treated with the following except:

A. Albuterol

B. Salmaterol

C. Propranolol

D. Salbutamol

(**EXPLAINATION:** Propranolol is a medication of the beta blocker type. It is used to treat high blood pressure, a number of types of irregular heart rate, thyrotoxicosis, capillary hemangiomas, performance anxiety, and essential tremors. It is used to prevent migraine headaches, and to prevent further heart problems in those with angina or previous heart attacks.)

75. Peg cell are seen in?

A. Vagina

B. vulva

C. ovary

D. Uterine tube

(**EXPLANATION:** A peg cell is a non-ciliated epithelial cell within the uterine tube (oviduct or

Fallopian tube). It is also called an "intercalary" cell or "secretory" cell. It is one of the two epithelial cells of the fallopian tube, along with ciliated simple columnar epithelial cells.

These cells produce a fluid that is rich in nutrients for spermatozoa, oocytes, and zygotes. The cellular secretions also promote the capacitation of spermatozoa by removing glycoproteins and other molecules from their cell membranes. The cells are outnumbered by ciliated cells in the oviduct, though their number can increase in response to progesterone.)

76. Part of eye used during eye donation is?
A. Iris
B. Retina
C. Cornea
D. Cones

77. Which of the following signs and symptoms indicate salicylate toxicity?
A. Chest pain
B. Pink coloured urine
C. Slow pulse rate
D. Ringing in ears

78. Chancre is seen in?
a. AIDS
b. Gonorrhoea

c. Syphilis

D. Hepatitis

(EXPLAINATION: A chancre is a painless ulceration (sore) most commonly formed during the primary stage of syphilis. This infectious lesion forms approximately 21 days after the initial exposure to Treponema pallidum, the gram-negative spirochaete bacterium yielding syphilis.**)**

79. Kernig's sign is present in which disease condition?

A. Keratitis

B. Renal failure

C. Meningitis

D. Brain tumour

80. The adrenal glands:

A. Are located near the thyroid gland.

B. Are located near the kidneys.

C. Are regulated by the posterior pituitary.

D. Are regulated by the pancreas.

(EXPLANATION: The adrenal glands (also known as supra-renal glands) are endocrine glands that produce a variety of hormones including adrenaline and the steroids aldosterone and cortisol. They are found above the kidneys. Each gland has an outer cortex which produces steroid hormones and an inner medulla. The adrenal cortex itself is divided into three zones: zona glomerulosa, the zona fasciculata and the zona reticularis.

The adrenal cortex produces three main types of steroid hormones: mineralocorticoids, glucocorticoids, and androgens. Mineralocorticoids (such as aldosterone) produced in the zona glomerulosa help in the regulation of blood pressure and electrolyte balance. The glucocorticoids cortisol and corticosterone are synthesized in the zona fasciculata; their functions include the regulation of metabolism and immune system suppression. The innermost layer of the cortex, the zona reticularis, produces androgens that are converted to fully functional sex hormones in the gonads and other target organs. The production of steroid hormones is called steroidogenesis, and involves a number of reactions and processes that take place in cortical cells. The medulla produces the catecholamines adrenaline and noradrenaline, which function to produce a rapid response throughout the body in stress situations.)

81. In the human body, the red blood cells are produced in?
A. Liver
B. Voluntary Muscles
C. Pancreas
D. Bone marrow

(**EXPLAINATION:** Production of red blood cells is controlled by erythropoietin, a hormone produced primarily by the kidneys. Red blood cells start as immature cells in the bone marrow and after approximately seven days of maturation are released into the bloodstream.)

82. Which of the following organ act as a " blood bank"?
A. Kidney
B. Heart
C. Spleen
D. Liver

83. Which hormone is responsible for diabetes insipidus?
A. Insulin
B. Vasopressin
C. Glucagon
D. Aldosterone

(**EXPLAINATION**: Diabetes insipidus (DI) occurs when the kidneys cannot concentrate the urine normally, and a large amount of dilute urine is excreted. The amount of water excreted in the urine is controlled by antidiuretic hormone (ADH). ADH is also called vasopressin. ADH is produced in a part of the brain called the hypothalamus.)

84. Widal test is used to detect?
A. Malaria
B. Typhoid
C. AIDS
D. None of the above

(**EXPLAINATION:** Widal Test is an agglutination test which detects the presence of serum agglutinins (H and O) in patients serum with typhoid and paratyphoid fever. When facilities for culturing are not available, the Widal test is the reliable and can be of value in the diagnosis of typhoid fevers in endemic areas.)

85. Bell's palsy affects which cranial nerve?
A. Optic nerve (II Cranial nerve)
B. Occulomotor(III Cranial Nerve)
C. Trochlear (IV Cranial nerve)
D. Facial (VII Cranial nerve)

(**EXPLAINATION:** Bell's palsy is a form of facial paralysis resulting from a dysfunction of the cranial nerve VII (the facial nerve) causing an inability to control facial muscles on the affected side. Often the eye in the affected side cannot be closed.)

86. Infection of bone is known as?
A. Osteoporosis
B. Osteomyelitis

C. Osteomalacia

D. Cellulitis

87. Blood cancer is also called....?

A. Thalassaemia

B. Haemophilia

C. Leukaemia

D. Cyanosis

(**EXPLAINATION:** Leukemia, is a group of cancers that usually begin in the bone marrow and result in high numbers of abnormal white blood cells. These white blood cells are not fully developed and are called blasts or leukemia cells. Symptoms may include bleeding and bruising problems, feeling tired, fever, and an increased risk of infections. These symptoms occur due to a lack of normal blood cells. Diagnosis is typically made by blood tests or bone marrow biopsy.**)**

88. Name the disease caused by human papilloma virus:

A. herpes simplex

B. warts

C. herpes zoster

D. psoriasis

89. In 28 days human ovarian cycle, ovulation occurs on:

A. 1 day

B. 5 days
C. 14 days
D. 28 days

90. What is the full form of ELISA?
A. Enzyme lysis immune solutions activity
B. Enzyme linked immune sorbent assay
C. Enzyme linked immune integrated solution activity
D. Enzyme lysis immuno solution assay

91. The choice of drug for treatment of alcoholism is
A. Disulfiram
B. Acyclovir
C. Haloperidol
D. Clonidine

(**EXPLAINATION:** Disulfiram works by inhibiting the enzyme acetaldehyde dehydrogenase, which means many of the effects of a "hangover" are felt immediately after alcohol is consumed.
In the body, alcohol is converted to acetaldehyde, which is then broken down by aldehyde dehydrogenase. If the dehydrogenase enzyme is inhibited, acetaldehyde builds up and causes unpleasant effects. Disulfiram should be used in conjunction with counseling and support.)

92. **Benedict test in a urine sample is done for the detection of?**
A. acetone
B. glucose
C. bile salt
D. bile pigment

93. **Dick test done in which disease:**
A. Scarlet fever
B typhoid fever
C tuberculosis
D thypus fever

94. **Koplik's spot is seen during the prodromal stage in case of:**
A. Measles
B. Typhoid
C. Diphtheria
D. Whooping cough

95. **Wilson's disease is due to abnormal accumulation of:**
A. Chromium
B. Nickel
C. Cobalt
D. Copper

96. **Schilling test is for diagnosis of?**
A. Fatty acid malabsorption
B. caeliac disease

C. hodgkins disease

D. vitamin B 12 deficiency

97. " Ketones Test " in the urine is done for the diagnosing of?

A. Aids

B. Down Syndrome

C. Gout

D. Diabetes Mellitus

98. Calcium deficiency in the body can be found due to absence of:

A. Vitamin B1

B. Vitamin E

C. Vitamin C

D. Vitamin D

99. To assessing a clinic patient with a diagnosis of hepatitis A. Which of the following is the most likely route of transmission?

A. Sexual contact with an infected partner.

B. Contaminated food.

C. Blood transfusion.

D. Illegal drug use.

(**EXPLAINATION:** Hepatitis A is the only type that is transmitted by the fecal-oral route through contaminated food. Hepatitis B, C, and D are transmitted through infected bodily fluids)

100. Snellen chart is used to:
A. record a child's growth.
B. measure a patient's vision.
C. determine values in spirometry.
D. monitor vital signs.

ANSWER KEY (Test Your knowledge)

1.A, 2.C, 3.B, 4.B, 5.C, 6.B, 7.B, 8.D, 9.D, 10.C, 11.C, 12.A, 13.C, 14.D, 15.C, 16.B, 17.C, 18.A, 19.D, 20.D, 21.B, 22.C, 23.D, 24.B, 25.A, 26.C, 27.A, 28.B, 29.C, 30.C, 31.D, 32.A, 33.B, 34.C, 35.D, 36.A, 37.C, 38.D, 39.B, 40.A, 41.D, 42.D, 43.C, 44.C, 45.D, 46.A, 47.D, 48.D, 49.A, 50.A, 51.A, 52.A, 53.A, 54.C, 55.A, 56.B, 57.B, 58.A, 59.C, 60.D, 61.A, 62.B, 63.D, 64.A, 65.D, 66.D, 67.D, 68.B, 69.C, 70.B, 71.B, 72.D, 73.B, 74.C, 75.D, 76.C, 77.D, 78.C, 79.C, 80.B, 81.D, 82.C, 83.B, 84.B, 85.D, 86.B, 87.C, 88.B, 89.C, 90.B, 91.A, 92.B, 93.A, 94.A, 95.D, 96.D, 97.D, 98.D, 99.B, 100.B

TEST YOUR KNOWLEDGE UNANI ASPECT

1. Nigella sativa botanical name hai:
A. kundur
B. loban
C. kasni
D. Kalonji

2. sultan ul ashjaar is the mutradif of?
A. ajwaain kharrasani
B. darmuna turky
C. siras
D. abnoos

3. Aza-e-Asliya hai:
A. Lahem
B. Shahem
C. Aza e mufridah
D. both a & b

4. Which of the following statement about bile is correct?
A. Bile is a chemical that will emulsify fat within the liver
B. Bile is an enzyme that will digest fat within the small intestine
C. Bile is a chemical that will emulsify fat within the small intestine
D. none of these

5. Nabz k Asbabe makuma hai:
A. hawa
B. riyazat
C. qalb ki quwate haiwania
D. makulaat

6. In the first phase of warm (darje ibteda) the following group of drugs are recommended:
A. Radiaat
B. Muhallil
C. Mushilat
D. Muhammirat

7. Junde bedastar ki muddate hayat hai:
A. 5year
B. 10year
C. 15year
D. 20year

8. Liber continents lateeni naam hai:
A. firdausul hikmat
B. kitabul kulliyaat
C. al hawi
D. none

(**EXPLAINATION:** Firdausul hikmat written by Rabban tabri, latin name is PARADISE OF WISDOM & kitabul kulliyat written by Ibn e Rushd, latin name is COLLIGET).

9. In case of Abdominal colic this unani drug my be prescribed:

A. Dhatoorah
B. Suranjan
C. Turbud
D. Non of the above

(EXPLAINATION: Dhatoorah has anticholinergic property that is the reason of it is effective in case of Abdominal colic by verchu of parasympatholytic action)

10. In mein se kaun si dawa "Mushil-e-Salasa" kehlati hai?

A. Alu Bukhara
B. Turbud
C. Maweez Munnaqa
D. Garequn

11. Makhzan Ul Advia ke mussanif kaun hain?

A. Hkm Sikandar
B. Hkm Niyaz Ahmad Khan
C. Najmul Gani
D. None of these

12. Kisi bhi dawa ke badal ke liye sabse Aham cheez:

A. Mizaj
B. Juz-e-khas

C. Chemical constituents

D. Afal

13. Sarphoka ka Botanical naam kiya hai?

A. Ruta graveolans

B. Echinochloa crusgalls

C. Tephorsia purpurea

D. Trapa spinosa

14. Afyun ki Muddat-e- hayat:

A. 50 years

B. 60 years

C. 70 years

D. 80 year

15. Baalon ki hifaazat karne waali dawa konsi hai?

A. parsiyaoshan

B. aamla

C. balchad

D. sabhi

16. Makhzan ul Hikmat ke musannif ka naam kiya hai?

A. Hakeem Firoz Uddin

B. Ghulam Jilani

C. Ismail Jarjani

D. Hakim Sikandar

17. Salq is a type of:

A. Wound

B. Dry burn

C. Wet burn

D. None

18. Other name of humma-e-mufattira is?
A. Lasiqa
B. Gibb-e-daira
C. Gibb-e-lazima
D. Muaziba

19. Tiryaq arba ka juz nahi hai:
A. Habbul gaar
B. Murmaki
B. Juntiyana
D. Anzaroot

20. kaunn si dawa Afyun ki aadat ko door karne ke leaye istemal hoti hai:
A. hab e jadwar
B. joher e raskapoor
C. hab e shifa
D. both A and C

21. Huzaaz is the disease related to?
A. Teeth
B. Nails
C. Scalp
D. Gums

22. Skin is a organ...
A. Mufarrad
B. Murakkab
C. Raees
D. None

23. Irq-e-madani is a:
A. Kharva
B. Narva
C. Salaa
D. Qamal

24. Total maternal weight gain during pregnancy is about?

A. 12.5 kg
B. 11 kg
C. 8 kg
D. 15 kg

(**EXPLAINATION:** First trimester 1 kg second and third 5+5+1=11kg. Pregnancy weight gain : 11 Kg's DC Dutta's Textbook of Obstetrics (Hiralal Konar) 8th Edition... Page No : 57)

25. The Synonym of "Marchoba"?
A. Haliyoon
B. Haloon
C. Jaloon
D. Qualoon

(**EXPLAINATION:** The synonym of "Marchoba" is a Haloon Jameul Advia - Dr Abdul Bari Page no : 76)

26. Choose 1 Medicine which is related to Plant Source?

A. Gauodanti
B. LodhPathaani

C. Lajaward

D. Naushaadar

27. Qurooh e reham has associated with:
A. dam
B. balgham
C. safra
D. sauda

28. bawasir(piles) me mufid (useful)hai:
A-rasot(berberis vulgaris)
B-jadwar(delphinium denudatum)
C-khaksi(sisymbrium iori)
D-all

29. Imtila be hasbil quwa is related to

A. quality of humour
B. quantity of humor
C. both
D. None

30. Which one of the following is not a cause of Uqr(sterlity):

A. farbahi
B. insidad e fam e reham
C. takkul e unq ur reham
D. mailan ur reham

31. Local application of hanzal is best drug for:

A. bars ul ain
B. sil ul ain
C. hujooz ul ain
D. maa e akhzar

32. "sangh pushpi" kiska mutradif hai:

A. mameraan
B. chalmogra
C. bansah
D. joze hindi

33. 'ummusshayateen' kis marz ko khte hain:

A. sara safrawi
B. juzam
C. shara, urticaria
D. none

34. 'Chaalmogra' ka kon se juz istemal hota hai:

A. fruit
B. bark
C. gum
D. whole plant

35. Tashkhees e mizaj k liye ajnaas e ashra ka zikr kisne kiya?

A. Razi
B. Majoosi
C. Ibn sena
D. Maseehi

36. Waram is a Disease of.....?
A. Mufrad
B. Motadil
C. Morakkab
D. Saada

37. Inme se kon maadni advia nahi hai?
a. sang basri
b. sang jarahat
c. sang sarmahi
d. none

38. Hiran khuri kis source ki dava hai?
A. Haiwani
B. madni
C. nabati
D. None

39. Waqoof is called as:
A. Ibteda
B. Inhetat
C. Tazaiyyud
D. Inteha

(EXPLAINATION: is darja me waram intehaaei haalat par pahonch kar Rukk jata hai)

40. Shafaqulus kiski qisam hai:
A. Sahar
B. Sarsaam
C. Sara
D. Subat

41. Smallest cells of Blood is...?

A. kuriyate hamra

B. kuriyate baiza

C. aqrase damvia

D. None

42. Dalk is included in?

A. Asbab-e-zarooriya

B. Asbab-e-maddiya

C. Asbab-e-gair zarooriya

D. Asbab-e-tamamiya

43. qai muzir hai:

A. malenkhoolia

B. wajaul mafasil

C. warme meda

D. isterkha meda

44. How is sleep after taking mushil qawi?

A. mufid

B. mamnu

C. muzir

D. none

45. kis hazam ke bad ghiza is qabil hoti hai ki tamam aza ko ghiza fraham ho sake:

A. hazm medi

b hazm kabadi

c hazm urooqui

d hazm uzwi

46. The Types of Quwa Mudrika are..

A. 2

B. 4

C. 3

D. 5

47. saqeeroos is:

A. warm e ruf

B. warm e kabid

C. warm e salb

D. warm e tihal

48. Which organ has barid & ratab temperament?

A. brain

B. liver

C. heart

D. spleen

49. most barid after izam:

A. asab

B. ribat

C. kurri

D. hair

50. Urticaria appearing in night is called:

A. shira e safravi

B. shira e damvi

C. shira balghami

D. shira saudavi

51. Quwa khyal KA MAQAM HAI:

A. muqaddam dimag

B. muakhar dimag

C. mukammal dimag

D. mutawassit dimag

52. When safra admixed with balgham ghaleez then it is termed as:

A. safra muhiyya

B. safra mirra

C. Safra kurrasi

D. Safra zanjari

53. Another name for quwa e mudrika is:

A. hawase ashra

B. hawase khamsa

C. hawase sitta

D. Hawase arba

54. Most ghaleez type of balgham is:

A. mayi

B. jassi

C. mukhati

D. zujaji

55. kaifiyat arba related to:

A. buqrat

B. jalunus

C. giroh mashayeen

D. none

56. In which disease huqna is not useful:
A. ishal
B. qoolanj
C. tukhma
D. warm gurda

57. According to Ibn Sina the hararate badani is:
A. asmani ya atayi hararat
B. unsure hararat
C. asmani wa unsure hararat
D. None

58. who said that qai is beneficial?
A. asqalibus
B. desquridoos
C. erasitratus
D. none

(**EXPLANATION:** buqrat ne kaha hai ki hifz sehat ke liye har mah me do martaba qai karana chahiye)

59. Habbe ayarij is DOC for ishal of:
A. safra
B. sauda
C. balgham
D. all

60. Amal e kadah kiya jata hai:
A. fistula lacrimalis me
B. exopthalmos me
C. cataract me
D. glaucoma me

61. Type of su e mizaj mufrad are:

A. 2

B. 4

C. 8

D. 10

62. Allama nafis ne blood ko kis se tasbiya di hai:

A. pani se

B. angoor se

C. sahad se

D. doodh se

63. Which drug is not effective in menorrhagia?

A. geru

B. dammul akhwaim

C. kaharba

D. sana makki

64. qawi way of istefragh is:

A. qai

B. ishal

C. fasad

D. tareeq

65. In all creature most motadil mizaj of:

A. human

B. animal

C. plants

D. aquatic plants

66. Which one of following is from falasafa e mashayeen?

A. arastu

B. buqrat

C. jalinus

D. Ibn sina

67. kanji is synonym of:

A. mari

B. abkama

C. sirka hindi

D. all

68. Fuqa is made from:

A. jau

B. khajoor

C. angoor

D. all

(**EXPLAINATION**: Jau ki Sharaab ko kahte hai)

69. Kaun sun stroke ka mutradif nhi hai:

A. zarbatus shams

B. subara

C. sakta e shamshiya

D. Huroor

70. Jalinoos ke nazdeek sura epilepsy ki wajah hai:

A. Ghaleez riyah

B. Ritubat-e-dimag

C. Dimag ki aziyat

D. Ghaleez khilt se paida shuda asbaab

(EXPLAINATION: Rutubat-e dimag BY Buqrat. Aziyat e dimag BY sheikh.

Ghaliz riyah BY Arastoo)

71. The seat of Quwa Shokia is ..

A. Dimagh

B. Nukha

C. Asb Hissi

D. Asb Hirki

72. Which quwa changes ghiza into johar e aza?

A. masika

B. hazima

C. dafia

D. jaziba

73. Asabe hissiya give khidmate .... to dimagh:

A. muhiyya

B. muwaddiya

C. zarooria

D. ghair zarooria

74. Dukkhan is:

A. Akhlat raddiya

B. hawa muheet

C. fuzlate rooh

D. none

75. Who compared rooh with chiraghe bairuni?
A. Buqrat
B. Ibn Sina
C. Ibn Zakariya
D. Sahibe Kamil

76. According to Abu Sahel Masihi lahm and shahm are also made from:
A. khoon
B. balgham
C. mani
D. Laban

77. What is useful in ikhtenaqur raham:
A. abzan
B. nutul
C. shamoom
D. ghusul

78. Muddirate bol are useful in:
A. Istisqa
B. falij
C. wajaul mafasil
D. all

79. according to Ibn Sina nuzj is required in which diseases:
A. amraze had
B. amraze muzmin
C. both
D None

80. Which of the following are Mudirrate harra?
A. parshiyaoshan
B. badyan
C. khubbazi
D. All

81. Which of the following are Mudirrate barida?
A. tukhm khyarain
B. tukhm khurfa
C. tukhm kasni
D. all

82. According to Jalinus nuzj is required in which diseases:
A. amraze had
B. amraze muzmin
C. amraze mufrida
D. all

83. Zarooni means zar i.e golden in colour it is a type of Majoon. The other meaning of zar is:
A. jad / stem
B. leaves
C. buds
D. Seeds

84. Safoof" MAJOOSI" Use kerte hain:
A. Niqras (gout)
B. HTN
C. Atherosclerosis
D. None

85. safoof bars k juz nahi hai:
A.babchi
B.panwad
C.injeer zerd
D.filfilseyah

86. "kaboos" hai:
A.malenkholiya ki qism
B.dabochne wala merz
C.unani tabeeb
D.none

(**EXPLAINATION:** Kaboos ko zaghoot bhi kahte hai, Nightmare. neend me ghutna yani dabochne wala marz.)

87. "Ye merz zameen k zalzala k manind h jo dafatan paida hota ar dafatan khtm ho jata hai"
A.saraa
B.falij
C.daur-raqs
D.all

88. "Billi lotan" hai:
A.badrunjaboya
B.qust talkh
C.Uood saleeb
D.none

89. Synonym of khibta is:
A. suda e har kharji
B. suda e barid dakhli

C. suda e barid kharji

D. suda e har dakhli

90. Jahuz is a disease of:

A. ears

B. eyes

C. nose

D. brain

91. Cardiac Arrest may be caused by:

A. Nux vomika

B. Digitalis

C. Abrus precatorius

D. opium

92. Road poison is:

A. Dhatura

B. Castor

C. Croton

D. Nux Vomika

93. Dammul Akhwain is:

A. resin of a plant

B. bark of a plant

C. root of a plant

D. none

94. Examples of Sui poison:

A. Abrus precatorius

B. Dhatura

C. Opium

D. all

95. kitab us saidana is authored by:
A. Rabban Tabari
B. Ibn Sina
C. Al Majoosi
D. Al Biruni

96. Humma reewiya kis fever ko kahte hai?
A. matbaqah ufoonia
B. sonukhas
C. matbaqah daaera
D. humma mawaziba

97. safrawi fever me behtareen ghiza:
A. mau-sh shaeir
B. maul-asl
C. kashkush shaeir
D. all

98. sadar kiska muqadma hai?
A. dwar ka
B. subaat ka
C. qoma ka
D. sarsam ka

99. tafsheel kya hai:
A. diet
B. medicine
C. vertigo me mufeed hai
D. All

100. Mirrah safra and safra muhaiya differ in:
A. colour
B. odour
C. viscosity
D. None

101. Tukm e turb is:
A. raphanus sativus
B. citrullus vulgaris
C. cucumis melo
D. none

102. Sayyal Advia ko injection k through jism me dakhil krne ka amal kahlata hai:
A. talqeeh
B. ehteqaan
C. sabig
D. all of above

(EXPLAINATION: Talqeeh vaccine ko kahte hai , vaccination ko amal talkeeh ya agr isse ilaj mansoob ho to ilaj bil talkeeh. ehteqaan (injection).

103. How many types of advia nabatiya?
A. 9
B. 10
C. 11
D. 12

104. Jalinoos al arab is the title of..
A. raazi
B. sheikh

C zohravi

D. jalinoos

105. According to `jalinoos` how many causes of "wajah"?

A. 5

B. 10

C. 15

D. 20

106. Hammam e ramli:

A. sand bath

B. acid bath

C. medicated bath

D. borax bath

107. Cupping is contraindicated in:

A. hummiyat

B. sara

C. in obese

D. all

108. How many types of rasoob gair tabyi?

A. 5

B. 6

C. 7

D. 8

109. Mahhjima is:

A. equipment of cupping

B. person who perform cupping

C. person whom cupping is performed

D. none

110. Which disease is related to baraze abyaz:

A. istesqa lahmi

B. yarqan suddi

C. baraze middi

D. yarqaane aswad

111. Gule seuti is also known as;

A. Gule nasreen

B. Gule mushkeen

C. Both a & b

D. None of the above

112. Jawasees -e dimagh hai:

A. hawase khamsa zahira

B. hawase khamsa batina

C. both

D. none

113. Artery ka nam kis basis par rakha gaya hai:

A. akhlat

B. rooh

C. quwa

D. none

114. Which process is used in the formation of kailoos?

A. istehala haqeeqiya

B. inqlab jauhari

C. both
D. none

115. Kis atibba ne kaha hai ki aazae raeesa 4 hai:
A. jalinoos
B. buqrat
C. Ibn sena
D. nafees

116. Hamil rooh urooq kahte hai:
A. vein
B. artery
C. nerve
D. a&b

117. The term Humujate medi is given by:
A. maseehi
B. hunain bin ishaque
C. ibn sena
D. nafees

118. Total no. of dalaile bol are:
A. 3
B. 5
C. 7
D. 9

119. Miqdar is included in:
A. adalla nabz
B. adalla bol
C. adalla baraz
D. all

120. Motadil jins of bol asfar is:
A. tibni
B. utraji
C. ashqar
D. ahmar nase

121. Kitabul illul aaraz ke musannif:
A. jalinoos
B. in sena
C. buqrat
D. ajmal khan

122. Color of rusube mahmood is:
A. asfar
B. abyaz
C. aswad
D. ahmar

123: Why fasd is a istefragh e kulli because:
A. it is used in all amraz
B. it do the istefragh of all akhlat
C. it evacuate all mawad from body
D. all

124. Chief ingredient of marhame e siyah is:
A. zangar
B. raal
C. murdar sang
D. shingarf

125. AKhlat are found in:
A. Urooq

B. Tafaveafe Badan

C. Tajaveefo Aza

D. Jiger

126. Musakkin tanaffus hai:

A. kushta karnullail

B. podina khushk

C. jund bedsatar

D. mastagi

127. Plants contain xanthotoxin:

A. afsanteen

B. atrilal

C. anhal

D. abresham

128. Drugs is of hot temperament:

A. luffah

B. shukran

C. tamar hindi

D. none

129. Farfeeran is synonym of:

A. Afyun

B. Farfiyun

C. Usara Revand

D. Usara Rasaut

130. Antidote hai:

A. anoshdaru

B. barshasha

C. dyaquza

D. none

131. Paneer maya nafe hai:
A. mirgi me
B. zof e qalb wa dimagh me
C. sailanurreham me
D. all

132. Todri hai:
A. tukhm
B. phool
C. jarh
D. gond

133. Qurs musallas ka nafe khas hai:
A. shaheeqa me
B. shaqeeqa me
C. wazaul fawad me
D. none

134. Following is example of Mizaj e Sani Gair Mustahkam Rikhu ba ifrat:
A. Baboona
B. Barg e kasni
C. Adas Musallam
D. All

135. Maulzehab ki prepration me shamil nahi hai:
A. pani
B. tezab namak
C. tezab shura
D. garam krna

136. Meaning of munaqqa:
A. Roasted
B. Cleaned and purified
C. Boiled
D. Pounded

137. Anushdaru ka juzae azam:
A. halela zard
B. aamla
C. bihi
D. baheda

138. tibbi maqsad ke liye ma'ul jaban behtar hota hai:
A. bakri ka
B. oont ka
C. gadhi ka
D. gaai ka

139. "FARANITUS" is:
A. sarsam-e-damvi
B. sarsam-e-balghmi
C. sarsam-e-safravi
D. none

140. Muqawwi basar is:
A. Feeroza
B. ood
C. tabasheer
D. kuchla

141. Muzir rehem hai:
A. haldi
B. aamla
C. abrak
D. farfyun

142. Gulqand is:
A. jamid
B. sayyal
C. neem jamid
D. none

143. Ufunat for bukhar is:
A. Sabab Kahrji
B. Sabab wasil
C. Sabab Zati
d. Sabab arzi

144. FAJALAT is mentioned under the heading of:
A. Murattibat
B. Mubarridat
C. Mujaffifat
D. Musakhinat

145. Hammam is a term used for:
A. Ek Jagah
B. Ek dawai ka naam hai
C. Ek Marz hai
D. Ghusl ko kahte hai

146. Component of water for Hammam Qabiz:
A. Darhald

B. Nakhoona
C. Baboona
D. Phitkari

147. Types of Asbabe kulliya are:
A. 2
B. 3
C. 4
D. 5

148. Marwareed ka badal hai:
A. Turbud
B. Rewand
C. Sadaf
D. All

149. Jali Advia ki shinakht kijeye:
A. Khardal
B. Namak
C. Both
D. None

150. Diyaqooza aor Abkama hai:
A. Jamid
B. Neem jamid
C. Bukhari
D. Sayyal

151. Markaze Bah hai:
A. Asab
B. Dimagh
C. Nukha

D. All

152. ILQA is a word used for:
A. Imagination by patient
B. Imagination by Hkm
C. Experiment by Hkm
D. Experiment by patient

153. Mushile zaeef hai:
A. Jamal goa
B. Sana makki
C. Turbud
D. All

154. Synonym for AADAT is:
A. Tabiyate oola
B. Tabiyate sania
C. Tabiyate salisa
D. None

155. Raqeeq baraz may be due to results of:
A. Zofe quwa jaziba
B. Zofe quwa masika
C. Zofe quwa hazima
D. All

156. Baraz ka tabayi rang hota hai:
A. Zard ma'il ba nariyat
B. Abyaz ma'il ba nariyat
C. Safed ma'il ba saudaviat
D. None

157. The color of baraz is due to:

A. Dam

B. Balgham

C. Safra

D. Sauda

158. Dala'ile Bol hai:

A. 3

B. 5

C. 7

D. 10

159. "Raeha bol" is used for:

A. Qiwam of qaroora

B. Color in qaroora

C. Reeh in qaroora

D. Bu in qaroora

160. Nabz Doodi inmei se kis se match khati hai:

A. Nabz moji

B. Nabz minsari

C. Nabz ghazali

D. All of the above

161. The pulse of moist temperament is:

A. small and slow

B. rapid and hard

C. hard and narrow

D. wide and wavy

162. The statement that "the increase of innate heat in the body leads to a corresponding decrease in strength" is:
A. true
B. not true
C. sometimes true
D. None of the above

163. In elderly people the pulse is:
A. small, slow and soft
B. small, rapid and soft
C. large, rapid and hard
D. large, slow and soft

164. causes of intermittent pulse:
A. great exhaustion
B. sudden disturbance
C. both
D. none

165. Distension caused by reeh is differentiated from other swellings by the:
A. pain caused by it
B. size of the swelling
C. shape of the swelling
D. amount of pressure required to overcome the tension

166. khyalat is a:
A. Dysfunction
B. Impairment

C. Loss of function
D. All

167. Twitching of the lower lip indicates:
A. Vomiting
B. Abdominal pain
C. Facial paralysis
D. Anxiety

168. Congenitally weak body organs are:
A. Liver and heart
B. Lungs and brain
C. Liver and kidney
D. All

169. Vital force (rooh) is a cause of weakness of organs due to its:
A. Abnormal temperament
B. Dispersion
C. Both
D. None

170. Abnormal humours cause pain by their:
A. Quality
B. Quantity
C. Both
D. None

171. Pain is not relieved by:
A. Heat
B. Cold
C. Moisture

D. All of the above

172. According to Galen, which is/are the real cause(s) of pain:

A. Imbalance of temperament

B. Imbalance of functions

C. Breach of continuity

D. All of the above

173. The causes of ulceration (taqarrah) are:

A. Sepsis in a wound

B. Rupture of matured swelling

C. Abcess eroding the adjoining tissues

D. All

174. Alate hawas indicates for:

A. Hawase khamsa

B. Aza nafsania

C. Khidmat imsak

D. Dimag wa nukh'a

175. "Sush" is included in:

A. Aza nafsania

B. Aza Haiwaniya

C. Aza tabaiya

D. Aza tanasuliya

175. Vehicle for ROOH is:

A. Dam

B. Balgham

C. Safra

D. Sauda

176. Causes of dislocation (khala) and displacement (mufarqat) are:
A. Moistening factors
B. Relaxing factors
C. Both
D. None

177. Abul arwah is the name used for:
A. Erasitratus
B. Jalinoos
C. Buqrat
D. None

178. Hulimate mukhandiqa is concern with:
A. Tongue
B. Hearing
C. Smell
D. Thought

179. Coitus (jimaa) produces:
A. Heat
B. Cold
C. Dryness
D. Moisture

180. Delayed staying in hot baths and undue retention of excretions produces:
A. Heat
B. Cold
C. Dryness
D. Moisture

181. Which type of cupping produces heat:
A. Wet cupping
B. Dry cupping
C. Both
D. None

(**EXPLAINATION**: DO'S AND DONT'S OF CUPPING THERAPY (Ref: Al- Qanun Fit tib. Canon of medicine (1025)

Dry cupping: Produces heat

Wet Cupping is considered as 'cooling' because it is considered to 'remove heat from the body'.

Nursing mothers: for scanty milk 'apply gentle dry cupping under the breasts'

Excessive menstrual bleeding: apply dry-cupping to the breasts, because blood tends to travel towards its related organ.

Wet cupping is contraindicated when there is blood deficiency "vacuousness"

Do not always bleed: It may prove sufficient to draw material away without actually evacuating.

To warm the skin: Apply dry cupping

Tightness and pain under the hypochondrium: Apply dry cupping with fire to the stomach region.

Avoid bleeding cupping: during fever that is accompanied by wasting.

After bathing: wait an hour before cupping

Infants: One should not begin to apply cupping to infants until they are in their third year.

Stomach pain: To allay pain apply over the umbilicus, cupping relives violent colic and flatulent distension of the abdomen and the uterine pain due to movement of the menstrual fluid, especially in young women.)

182. Mechanism of wet cupping therapy (Hijama) is dominated by control in:

A. Neural

B. Haematological

C. Immune system functioning

D. All of the above

(**EXPLAINATION:** Mechanism of wet cupping is dominated by control in NEURAL, HAEMATOLOGICAL, and IMMUNE SYSTEM FUNCTIONING.

Main effects wct may occurs as , (1) irritation of the immune system by producing local simulated inflammation followed by activation of complementary system and increase level of immune products such as interferon and tumor necrotizing fators, and (2) organize of traffic of lymph and an increase in the flow of lymph in lymph vessels, (3) and effect on thymus. (4) In the neural system effects occurs by regulation of neurotransmitters and hormones like serotonin , dopamine, endorphin , acetylcholine etc.

In the haematological system, main effects occurs by these two pathways: (i) regulation of coagulation and anti-coagulation systems like decrease in the level of haematological element such as fibrinogen (ii) decrease n the hematocrit, followed by increase in the blood flow and in the end organ oxygenation)

183. Injezabe safra occurs in:
A. Duodenum
B. Ilium
C. Large intestine
D. All of the above

184. Sarira and Jahira are the types of:
A. Dam
B. Balgham
C. Safra
D. Sauda

185. Madda quwa hai:
A. Arwah wa akhlat
B. Akhlat wa mizaj
C. A'za wa af'al
D. all of the above

186. Raddi fuzla nahi hai:
A. Arq
B. Bol
C. Baraz
D. Mani

187. Concept of Halat salisa was given by:
A. Jalinoos
B. Razi
C. Ibn Sina
D. Ibn Baitar

188. Which one water beneficial effects for spleen:
A. Ma; nuhasia
B. Ma' hadeedia
C. Both
D. None

189. Which one is correct term?
A. Istefragh Juzwi
B. Istefragh Jussi
C. Istefragh Uzwi
D. None of the above

190. Rua'f is:
A. Ehtabas
B. Istefragh
C. Harkat badania
D. All of the above

191. Which bath having beneficial effects in cleanses the uterus?
A. Water bath
B. Oil bath
C. Sand bath
D. Sun bath

192. "Mahafa" is a term used for:
A. A especially equipped bed
B. A specially equipped stretcher
C. A specially equipped vehicle
D. A specially equipped room

193. Summer (saif) turns the complexion:
A. red
B. pink
C. yellow
D. blue

194. Sehat ke liye zaroori hai:
A. Ehtbas
B. Istefragh
C. Balance between Ehatbas wa istefragh
D. All of the above

195. Musariat is a type of riyazat:
A. Kushti ladna
B. Tez chalna
C. Kashti chalana
D. None

196. The predisposing (sabiqa) cause of glaucoma is the:
A. general excess of humours (ghalba-e-akhlat)
B. putrefaction of humours (fasaad-e-akhlat)
C. both
D. none

197. Quwwat-e- haiwania is located in:
A. liver
B. heart
C. kidney
D. brain

198. Use of munzijat , before using mushily is:
A. Zaroori hai
B. Ghair zaroori hai
C. Should not be given
D. All are correct

199. Mushil den eke liye sabse acha season hai:
A. Rabi
B. Khareef
C. Shita
D. Khiza

200. Zayeqa ke aitbaar se balgham ghair tabayi ki qisme hai:
A. 2
B. 4
C. 5
D. 6

ANSWER KEY (Test your knowledge Unani Aspect)

1.D, 2.C, 3.B, 4.C, 5.C, 6.A, 7.B, 8.C, 9.A, 10.D, 11.C, 12.A, 13.C, 14.A, 15.B, 16.B, 17.C, 18.B, 19.D, 20.D, 21.C, 22.A, 23.B, 24.B, 25.B, 26.B, 27.C, 28.A, 29.B, 30.C, 31.A, 32.C, 33.A, 34.A, 35.D, 36.C, 37.C, 38.C, 39.D, 40.B, 41.A, 42.C, 43.C, 44.A, 45.B, 46.A, 47.C, 48.A, 49.B, 50.C, 51.A, 52.A, 53.A, 54.B, 55.C, 56.C, 57.A, 58.D, 59.D, 60.C, 61.B, 62.B, 63.D, 64.B, 65.A, 66.A, 67.D, 68.A, 69.B, 70.D, 71.A, 72.B, 73.A, 74.C, 75.D, 76.A, 77.A, 78.D, 79.C, 80.D, 81.D, 82.B, 83.D, 84.A, 85.D, 86.B, 87.A, 88.A, 89.C, 90.B, 91.B, 92.A, 93.A, 94.A, 95.D, 96.A, 97.A, 98.A, 99.A, 100.C, 101.A, 102.B, 103.C, 104.A, 105.C, 106.A, 107.D, 108.D, 109.A, 110.B, 111.C, 112.A, 113.B, 114.C, 115.A, 116.B, 117.B, 118.C, 119.D, 120.B, 121.A, 122.B, 123.B, 124.B, 125.A, 126.A, 127.B, 128.D, 129.C, 130.B, 131.D, 132.A, 133.B, 134.B, 135.D, 136.B, 137.B, 138.A, 139.A, 140.A, 141.D, 142.C, 143.B, 144.B, 145.A, 146.D, 147.B, 148.C, 149.C, 150.D, 151.C, 152.A, 153.B, 154.B, 155.D, 156.A, 157.C, 158.C, 159.C, 160.A, 161.D, 162.B, 163.A, 164.C, 165.D, 166.A, 167.A, 168.B, 169.C, 170.C, 171.A, 172.C, 173.D, 174.A, 174.B, 175.A, 176.C, 177.A, 178.A, 179.C, 180.B, 181.B, 182.D, 183.A, 184.C, 185.A, 186.D, 187.A, 188.C, 189.A, 190.B, 191.D, 192.B, 193.C, 194.C, 195.A, 196.A, 197.B, 198.A, 199.A, 200.B

OTHER MCQ'S BOOKS FOR PREPARATION THE PH.D, PG AND MO UNANI EXAMINATIONS.

1. The Prime: Mcqs for Post Graduation Unani Entrance Examination by Dr Izharul Hasan & Dr Haqeeq Ahmad

(Available on all AMAZON Stores online)

THIS BOOK COVERS THE FOLLOWING EXAMINATION SOLVED PAPERS:

1 RAJASTHAN UNANI MEDICAL OFFICER 2011 (9-18)
2 RAJASTHAN UNANI MEDICAL OFFICER 2012 (19-27)
3 MADHYA PRDESH UNANIMEDICALOFFICER 2013 (28-37)
4 CHHATISH GARH UNANI MEDICAL OFFICER 2009 (38-47)
5 JUMM UNANI MEDICAL OFFICER 2009 (48-56)

6 JAMMU & KASHMIR UNANI MEDICAL OFFICER 2012 (57-68)
7 CHENNAI UNANI MEDICAL OFFICER PAPER 2011 (69-79)
8 CHENNAI UNANI MEDICAL OFFICER 2012 (80-90)
9 UNNAI MEDICAL OFFICER MODEL PAPER ONE (91-100)
10 UNNAI MEDICAL OFFICER MODEL PAPER TWO (101-111)
11 UNNAI MEDICAL OFFICER MODEL PAPER THREE (112-121)
12 TEST YOUR KNOWLEDGE ONE (AMRAZ E NISWAN WA QABALAT) (122-132)
13 TEST YOUR KNOWLEDGE TWO (ANATOMY, PHYSIOLOGY & BIOCHEMISTRY) (133-143)
14 TEST YOUR KNOWLEDGE THREE (ILMUL ADVIA) (144-154)
15 TEST YOUR KNOWLEDGE FOUR (KULLIYAT) (155-165)
16 TEST YOUR KNOWLEDGE FIVE (MOALIJAT) (166-175)
17 TEST YOUR KNOWLEDGE SIX (MOALIJAT) (176-185)
18 TEST YOUR KNOWLEDGE SEVEN (ILMUL ADVIA) (186-195)
19 TEST YOUR KNOWLEDGE EIGHT (SURGERY AND REGIMENTAL THERAPY) (196-206)
20 TEST YOUR KNOWLEDGE NINE (TAHAFFUJI WA SAMAJI TIBB) (207-218)
21 TEST YOUR KNOWLEDGE TEN (REVISION-1) (219-229)
22 TEST YOUR KNOWLEDGE ELEVEN (REVISION-II) (230-239)
23 TEST YOUR KNOWLEDGE TWELVE (REVISION-III) (240-250)

24 MD UNANI ENTRANCE EXAM NIUM 2005 (251-260)
25 MD UNANI ENTRANCE EXAM NIUM 2006 (261-270)
26 MD UNANI ENTRANCE EXAM NIUM 2007 (271-280)
27 MD UNANI ENTRANCE EXAM NIUM 2008 (281-290)
28 MD UNANI ENTRANCE EXAM NIUM 2009 (291-300)
29 MD UNANI ENTRANCE EXAM NIUM 2010 301-310
30 MD UNANI ENTRANCE EXAM NIUM 2011 (311-319)
31 MD UNANI ENTRANCE EXAM NIUM 2012 (320-328)
32 MD UNANI ENTRANCE EXAM NIUM 2013 (329-336)
33 MD UNANI ENTRANCE EXAM NIUM 2014 337-344
34 MD EXAM UNANI ENTRANCE (DU) 2009 345-352
35 MD EXAM UNANI ENTRANCE (DU) 2010 (353-360)
36 MD EXAM UNANI ENTRANCE (DU) 2011 (361-368)
37 MD EXAM UNANI ENTRANCE (DU) 2012 (369-376)
38 MD EXAM UNANI ENTRANCE (DU) 2013 (377-384)
39 MD UNANI ENTRANCE EXAM HYDERABAD 2012 (385-391)
40 MD UNANI ENTRANCE EXAM HYDERABAD 2012 (392-398)

2. The Premier, Previous Examination Papers of MD Unani Amu Aligarh: Mcq 2200 With Answers Key by Dr Izharul Hasan & Dr Haqeeq Ahmad

(Available on all AMAZON Stores online)

THIS BOOK COVERS THE FOLLOWING EXAMINATION SOLVED PAPERS:

1. MD Unani AMU ENTRANCE EXAMNATION 2014-15(6-45)
2. MD Unani AMU ENTRANCE EXAMNATION 2013-14 (46-84)
3. MD Unani AMU ENTRANCE EXAMNATION 2012-13 (85-122)
4. MD Unani AMU ENTRANCE EXAMNATION 2010-11 (123-160)
5. MD Unani AMU ENTRANCE EXAMNATION 2009-10 (161-198)
6. MD Unani AMU ENTRANCE EXAMNATION 2006-07 (199-241)
7. MD Unani AMU ENTRANCE EXAMNATION 2005-06 (242-283)

8. MD Unani AMU ENTRANCE EXAMNATION 2004-05 (284-321)
9. TEST YOUR KNOWLEDGE (MODEL 1) JARAHAT & TST (322-364)
10. TEST YOUR KNOWLEDGE (MODEL 2) AMRAZE-NISWAN & MOALIJAT (365-406)
11. TEST YOUR KNOWLEDGE (MODEL 3) ADVIA AND KULIYAT (407-444)

www.ingramcontent.com/pod-product-compliance
Lightning Source LLC
Chambersburg PA
CBHW071412180526
45170CB00001B/87